KETO AFTER 50

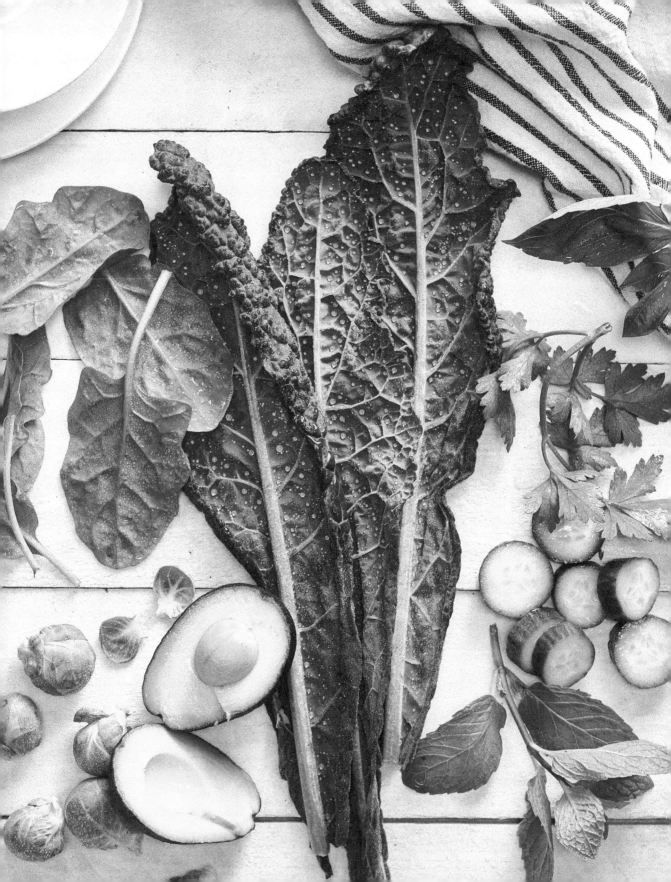

KETO AFTER 50

A Complete Plan for Staying Healthy, Eating Well, and Losing Weight

MOLLY DEVINE, RD

ROCKRIDGE
PRESS

For general information on our other products and services or to obtain technical support, please contact our Customer Care Department within the United States at (866) 744-2665, or outside the United States at (510) 253-0500.

Rockridge Press publishes its books in a variety of electronic and print formats. Some content that appears in print may not be available in electronic books, and vice versa.

TRADEMARKS: Rockridge Press and the Rockridge Press logo are trademarks or registered trademarks of Callisto Media Inc. and/or its affiliates, in the United States and other countries, and may not be used without written permission. All other trademarks are the property of their respective owners. Rockridge Press is not associated with any product or vendor mentioned in this book.

Interior and Cover Designer: Erin Yeung
Art Producer: Meg Baggott
Editor: Cecily McAndrews
Production Editor: Ashley Polikoff

Cover photograph © 2021 Annie Martin; Thomas J. Story, p. ii; Evi Abeler, p. vi, 132; Darren Muir, p. viii, 2; Cameron Whitman/Stocksy United, p. 12, 98; Nadine Greeff, p. 20; Sarka Babicka/Stockfood, USA, p. 48; Ewgenija Schall/Stockfood, USA, p. 66; Keller & Keller/Stockfood, USA, p. 80; Unzer Verlag/Maria Brinkop/Stockfood, USA, p 118

Author photo courtesy of Heba Salama Photography

ISBN: Print 978-1-64876-847-7
eBook 978-1-64876-848-4

R0

For all of my strong and beautiful patients;
I am so grateful to be a part of your health journey.

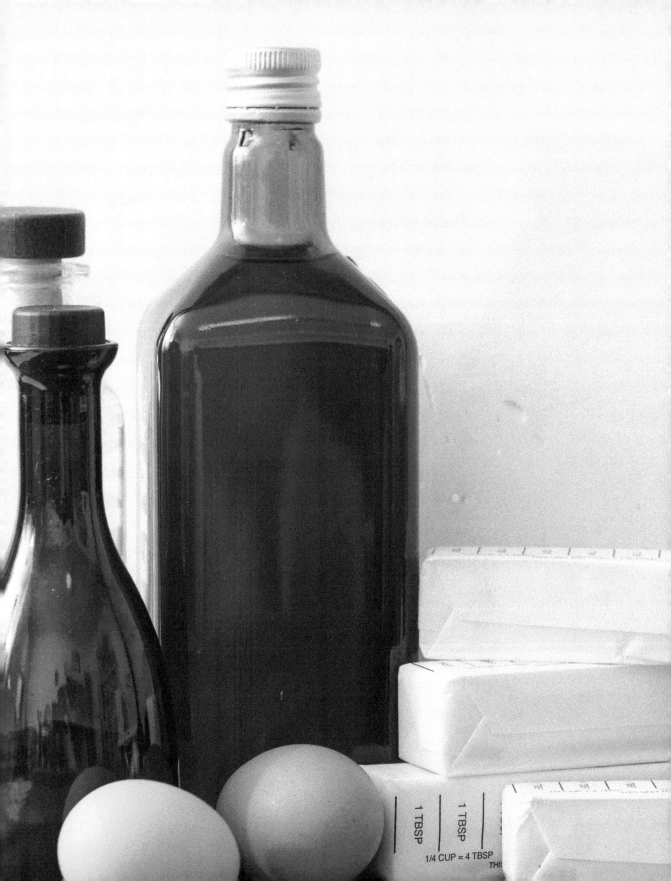

CONTENTS

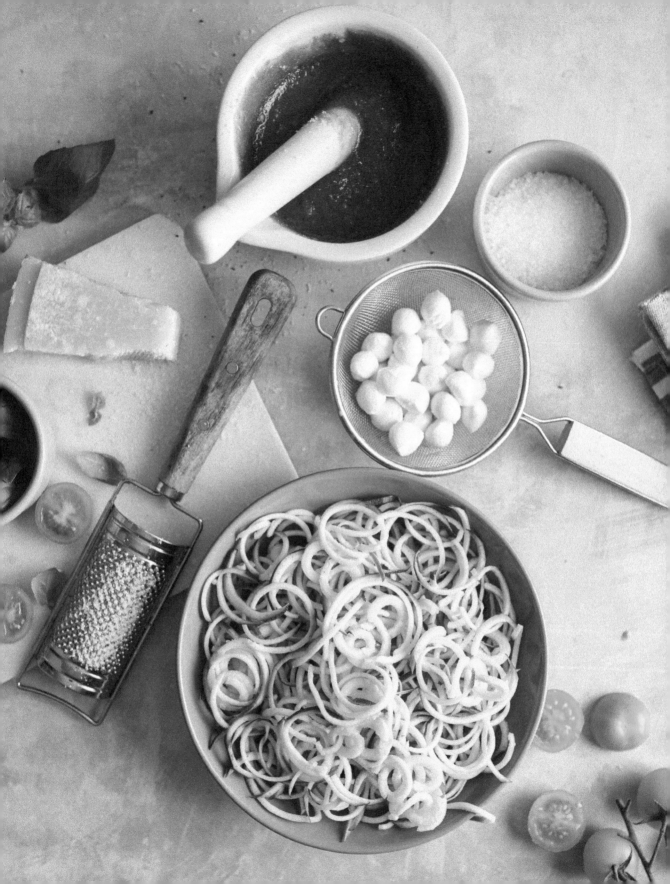

INTRODUCTION

As we age, a healthy lifestyle becomes more important than ever before. In my career as a registered and licensed dietitian, I have witnessed the power of quality nutrition and its positive impact on my patients' long-term health. I firmly believe that being mindful about the food we eat is the best way to drastically improve and enhance our quality of life.

I began implementing ketogenic nutrition therapy at my nutrition counseling practice after seeing firsthand how this way of eating can reduce inflammation, improve digestive health, and enhance energy and mental clarity. My patients are often amazed at how much better they feel, both physically and mentally, after changing their nutrition habits. In fact, many are able to get off prescription medications that they have been on for years. This heightened quality of life provides even more motivation, making a healthy high-fat/low-carbohydrate dietary approach very sustainable for the long term.

The keto diet has gained a wide audience in recent years for its many health benefits, including the ability to improve and often reverse many chronic conditions, including type 2 diabetes and neurological conditions such as Parkinson's and epilepsy. It is also an effective way to lose weight and improve body composition.

That said, not all ketogenic diets are created equal, and not all ketogenic diets are healthy in the long term. A well-formulated keto diet—one designed for lasting health benefits—does not mean "all the fats all the time." Many "dirty keto" approaches include inflammatory fats, insufficient levels of micronutrients from vegetables, and a high level of processed meats, which together can actually lead to negative health outcomes over time. The best way to approach the ketogenic diet (or really any diet) is with guidance and customization for specific age, gender, and health conditions.

Success begins with knowledge and a solid, doable plan. I wrote this book to provide you with both, as the meal plans and recipes in this book target the specific needs of people over 50.

In the first two chapters, I will help you understand your body's metabolic needs, and explain why it may react in certain ways to different foods. We'll explore what a good ketogenic diet consists of, as well as how to implement this approach, including a 28-day meal plan (chapter 3), and in the remaining chapters, 55 flavorful and nutrient-dense recipes.

I hope you come to enjoy the ketogenic lifestyle as much as I do, and that you find the health benefits inspirational for your continued, long-term success.

PART ONE

GOING KETO AFTER 50

Everybody is different: What may work wonderfully for a healthy 25-year-old man may not be the best approach for, say, a 55-year-old woman. Often, patients come to me frustrated after having started a ketogenic diet that they found on the Internet and not seeing results or feeling great. This doesn't mean that keto isn't for you—it just means that you haven't found the best keto approach for you.

I believe in the power and importance of educating yourself about nutrition, and a customized approach that addresses your unique needs for long-term success and sustainability. I want to empower you with valuable knowledge to help you understand how your nutrition needs change with age, set realistic expectations for progress, and achieve lasting results. If you are ready to find a nutrition and lifestyle plan that will positively impact your long-term health and make a clean ketogenic diet work for your needs, this is the book for you!

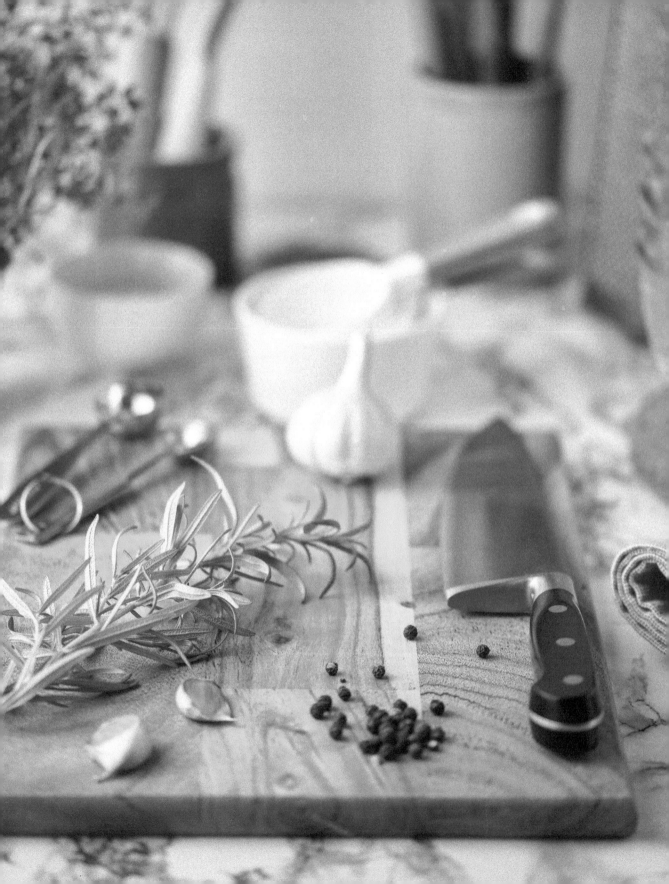

CHAPTER ONE

Keto for You

Proper nutrition is the universal foundation of a healthy lifestyle, but this becomes even more important as we age, for many reasons. The body's response to inflammatory foods such as sugars and refined carbohydrates is heightened with age, and can increase the risk of developing a chronic disease. While many younger keto dieters may solely focus on weight loss, those over 50 who look to this diet often have a broader focus on improving health and longevity while maintaining a healthy weight. I certainly understand that for many, seeing the scale go down can feel like a victory, but I reinforce with all my patients that weight loss is really just a (positive!) side effect of maintaining a healthy lifestyle, and isn't the most important goal. In this chapter, we'll explore the relationship between dietary choices and health as we age.

What Is the Ketogenic Diet and Why Should I Try It?

The CDC's "National Diabetes Statistics Report for 2020" found that just over one in ten Americans have type 2 diabetes and one in three Americans have prediabetes. They predict that by 2030, more than 15 percent of adult Americans will have type 2 diabetes. This staggering number reflects the harsh toll the Standard American Diet has taken. The Standard American Diet, also called SAD, is the name given to the typical diet followed by most Americans—high in refined carbohydrates, sugars, and processed foods—and is one of the leading causes of chronic disease in our country.

Type 2 diabetes, the deadly disease that is also the cause of many other complications, is 100 percent preventable through proper nutrition and dietary habits. The risk for developing diabetes increases significantly over the age of 45, making this life stage a vital time for positive dietary changes, including a very low-carb/high-healthy fat ketogenic diet.

Many people believe that a ketogenic diet is simply "low carb," but there's more to it. The majority of energy, or calories, consumed on a ketogenic diet comes from dietary fat. Only a moderate amount comes from protein, and a very low amount comes from carbohydrates. The body naturally prefers to burn glucose (from carbs), but when deprived of glucose, it turns to burning fat, relying on both dietary fat sources as well as stored body fat for energy. This is the metabolic state of *ketosis*, from which the ketogenic diet derives its name. In a state of ketosis, blood sugars decrease if they were elevated, and levels of circulating insulin decrease—this results in less fat storage and reduced inflammation.

WHAT ARE MACROS? WHY ARE THEY IMPORTANT?

Macronutrients, or *macros* for short, are the building blocks of our diet. They are the nutrients we need to function. All food breaks down into one of three (or a combination of the three) macros: protein, carbohydrates, and fat. To achieve and maintain a state of metabolic ketosis, you want the majority of calories in your diet to be derived from fat, a moderate amount from protein, and a bare minimum from carbohydrates. This will prevent spikes in glucose and insulin, and allow for ketone production from fat cells (ketosis).

Various lifestyle factors, such as sleep, stress, timing of meals, and exercise, can have a big impact on specific individual macronutrient ratios—both for maintaining ketosis and for weight loss (if that is your goal). Additionally, conditions such as diabetes and related insulin resistance may reduce the amount of dietary carbohydrates certain people can tolerate.

For long-term success on a ketogenic diet, you'll need to make modifications as you go for your individual needs, based on activity level, weight-loss goals, and hunger levels. However, I always start my clients out on a strict macronutrient ratio plan to induce ketosis as quickly as possible, diminish carb cravings, and spark improvements in energy levels, mental function, and body composition.

Specifically for people over 50, I recommend following a 70-20-10 ratio of fat-protein-total carbohydrate, keeping total carbs—not net—under 30g each day (see "What's the Story with Net Carbs?," page 18). This ratio is high enough in fat to help curb cravings and fill you up and adequate enough in protein for those over 50 who have increased needs with age. But it's not so high that it will prevent ketosis, and it's low enough in carbs to trigger immediate results. After an initial four- to six-week metabolic transition, some people can start to tweak their ratios by increasing nonstarchy vegetables or proteins without a reduction in ketone levels. However, refined carbohydrates, sugars, most grains, and starches will prevent a state of ketosis, as the body returns to burning its favored energy source: glucose.

WHAT IS KETOSIS?

When you stop supplying your body with glucose from carbohydrates, it will look for a new fuel source for energy and cell function. Not all cells can use pure fatty acids for fuel—most important, the brain cannot use them at all. Ketosis is the body's natural metabolic process of converting these fatty acids into usable currency for energy: ketones.

In ketosis, fatty acids travel to the liver, where they are converted into ketones and sent throughout the body for use as energy. Ketones are like rocket fuel: They are extremely efficient, provide long-term energy, and improve overall mental function.

The ability to achieve ketosis is different for everyone and varies based on previous carbohydrate intake, body composition, insulin resistance, and fitness level. But generally, following the strict ketogenic ratios and meal plans outlined in the following chapters should allow your body to enter ketosis within three to four days.

WHAT HAPPENS TO MY BODY ON KETO?

Once your body enters ketosis and starts to become increasingly efficient producing and using ketones as its primary fuel source, you can expect a reduction in hunger; an improvement in energy, mental clarity, and sleep; and a reduction in inflammation.

When your brain is consistently fueled by ketones and not glucose, it stops craving or looking for a steady stream of carbohydrate- and sugar-dense foods. This makes avoiding these foods easier. Additionally, brain function and mental energy improve drastically when fueled by the powerhouse ketones. You'll feel less hunger as your body adapts to utilizing stored energy (from body fat) for fuel between meals, making the need for snacking obsolete. For most people, it is the first time they don't feel hungry all the time on a diet!

What's Different About Keto After 50

Without a doubt, 50 is the new 40 or even 30! I remember as a child, my parents and their friends attending "over the hill" parties as their friends rounded the corner into the "dreaded" middle age.

Now as an adult, having long past rounded that corner myself and with a majority of my patients well into their fifties, sixties, and seventies, I no longer think of over 50 as old. In fact, it's an exciting opportunity, as now is the most important time in your life to make these healthy lifestyle changes so you can enjoy many vibrant years feeling good.

Aging does not have to result in developing diseases and popping lots of medications. You don't have to resign yourself to simply accepting a chronic condition; you often have the power to reverse it, get off medication, and feel energized again. Taking control of your health through proper nutrition and a well-formulated low-carb/high-healthy-fat ketogenic diet can add years to your life. Now is the time to stop being frustrated with your health and take control of your future!

NUTRITION AFTER 50

The effects of aging actually begin around age 30, when the human growth period draws to a close, and senescence, or the organic process of growing older and displaying the effects of increased age, begins. Factors such as genetics, illness, and lifestyle all play important roles in how aging progresses for each individual, but disease and reduced function are *not* an inevitable result of the aging process! Proper nutrition that focuses on the right amounts of macronutrients (proteins, carbohydrates, and fats) as well as micronutrients (vitamins and minerals), timing of meals, and activity levels can prevent many of the negative impacts of natural aging.

It is a fact that body composition changes as we age. Lean muscle mass decreases and fat mass and visceral fat around the abdomen increase. Sedentary lifestyles, combined with poor nutrition, accelerate this natural process, while more active individuals with better blood sugar control through proper dietary choices will be less impacted by this effect of aging.

The negative side effects of age-related obesity include:

» Type 2 diabetes
» Cardiovascular disease (CVD)
» Hypertension (high blood pressure)
» Arthritis
» Fatty liver disease

In fact, while CVD is the leading cause of death in the United States, it is not a disease of aging, but rather a nutrition-related disease stemming from unhealthy food choices over time.

Neurological health is another concern. While some memory decline is normal as we age, the likelihood and severity of conditions such as dementia, Alzheimer's disease, and Parkinson's disease can be increased by poor dietary choices. The ketogenic diet is being studied as a viable therapy in preventing and managing these degenerative neurological conditions, as ketones provide an optimal energy source for the brain, leading to improved mental function.

Since so many age-related conditions can be prevented through proper nutrition, a ketogenic diet can slow the signs of aging—but it's so important to make sure this also aligns with your specific needs and lifestyle as someone over the age of 50. Fat is the main source of energy in any ketogenic diet, but the *type* of fat is even more important as we age to maintain heart health and decrease inflammation. Saturated fats from animal sources are fine to include in moderation, but the majority of fats should come from unsaturated, heart-healthy fats, such as those found in olive oil, nuts, seeds, avocados, and fatty fish.

Similarly, the *quality* of your protein sources matter. Many older adults suffer from high blood pressure (hypertension), which can be exacerbated by an excessively high-sodium diet. Avoiding large quantities of highly processed meats such as deli meats, hot dogs, and bacon, and focusing on quality free-range and grass-fed meats, poultry, and eggs, as well as wild-caught seafood, helps to keep sodium levels in check and reduce inflammation.

Last, we can't forget about the micronutrients that are so important to overall health, especially as we age. Many "dirty keto" diets include unlimited quantities of poor-quality proteins and fats, and rely on processed and packaged keto products instead of colorful plants and berries as the main source of carbohydrates. These diets lack the essential fiber, vitamins, and minerals integral for bone, skin, metabolic, and digestive health, especially as we age.

Many people expect to see drastic weight loss when starting a ketogenic diet, but this is not necessarily the case for everyone, especially for those over 50. Metabolic function declines with age and loss of muscle mass; plus, for many women, hormonal shifts can impact insulin levels, making maintaining ketosis more difficult and weight loss much slower.

However, this should not deter anyone from adopting this lifestyle! The non-weight-related benefits of keto, such as reduced inflammation, improved mental health, increased energy, decreased sugar cravings, and improved lab results far outweigh daily scale victories. Weight loss is often a positive side effect of a healthy lifestyle, but may not be rapid for everyone.

For those with weight-loss goals, simply following ketogenic ratios and achieving ketosis does not automatically lead to weight loss. Calories are still important, especially as we age and metabolic rates decrease naturally. A state of ketosis just means using ketones (as fat) for fuel. These can come from dietary fats (what you put in your mouth) or stored body fats. In order to see weight loss on the scale, it's necessary to find the right balance of overall calories so your body will turn to its stored fat for some energy expenditure. The meal plans that follow are designed around varying calorie levels based on your individual size and gender, but all provide an optimal energy balance to promote nutritional ketosis along with improvements in body composition.

Benefits of Keto After 50

Emerging research shows the many benefits of a ketogenic diet, both for general health and for managing chronic diseases. Specifically for people over 50, a well-formulated ketogenic diet can help with:

Blood sugar control. Studies show that the reduced carbohydrate consumption in a ketogenic diet can reduce blood sugar and insulin fluctuations. Better insulin control and reversal of insulin resistance can help improve metabolic disorders like type 2 diabetes, as well as symptoms linked to high insulin and blood sugar.

Long-term cardiac health. For decades, we all heard that fat will not only make us fat, but that high-fat diets (particularly those high in saturated animal fats) are the main cause of heart disease. We are now learning that this does not represent the full picture. It is the combination of refined and processed carbohydrates and sugars along with a high intake of dietary fats that elevate triglycerides (fat molecules in the blood) and increase the concentration of unhealthy LDL cholesterol. Eating a good balance of the right type of healthy fats, while limiting carbohydrate intake, can improve the good HDL cholesterol levels and lower bad LDL cholesterol levels, reducing the risk for cardiac disease.

Neurological function. Aside from the positive psychological associations with improvements in health and physical function (specifically, improved mood and sleep), there is science behind the powers of a ketogenic diet on brain health. When the body is in ketosis, the brain utilizes ketones, a more efficient fuel source than glucose, which leads to feeling more alert and mentally energized throughout the day. The ketogenic diet is currently being studied for its potential beneficial impacts on other neurological diseases, such as Alzheimer's and Parkinson's disease.

Reduced joint inflammation (arthritis). Another well-studied benefit of a ketogenic diet is the production of high levels of anti-inflammatory adenosine during metabolism in ketosis. While complete reversal of arthritis is uncommon, many patients report a significant decrease in pain or need for medication to manage their pain.

Beyond helping the chronic conditions listed here, the ketogenic diet helps improve quality of life in a whole host of other ways:

» Improved sleep
» Improved hormonal balance
» Decreased occurrence of depressive thoughts
» Enhanced mood from better brain health and stable energy levels

Listen to Your Body and Talk to Your Doctor

These days, more medical professionals are accepting the ketogenic diet as a way to help patients manage and reverse many chronic diseases. However, some conditions may make following a high-fat ketogenic diet more difficult. Always discuss your personal health concerns with your doctor or a registered dietitian before implementing any medical nutrition therapy.

Conditions to consider include:

Cholecystectomy. If your gallbladder has been removed in the past six months, you will likely have difficulty digesting a high-fat diet and will need to be monitored for potential adverse side effects.

Renal disease. Individuals with chronic kidney disease or who suffer from chronic kidney stones may need to regulate their protein intake. As mentioned previously, a ketogenic diet is not a high-protein diet, but many people replace carbs with protein, which can overload ailing kidneys.

Insulin-dependent diabetes. Drastically reducing your carbohydrate intake will necessitate a change in your insulin dosage. Discuss your new dietary approach with your endocrinologist to help with this transition.

Hypertension. Reducing body weight by 5 to 10 percent can reverse hypertension naturally. If you are on blood pressure medication, be sure to monitor both blood pressure as well as weight with your doctor to avoid episodes of hypotension (low blood pressure).

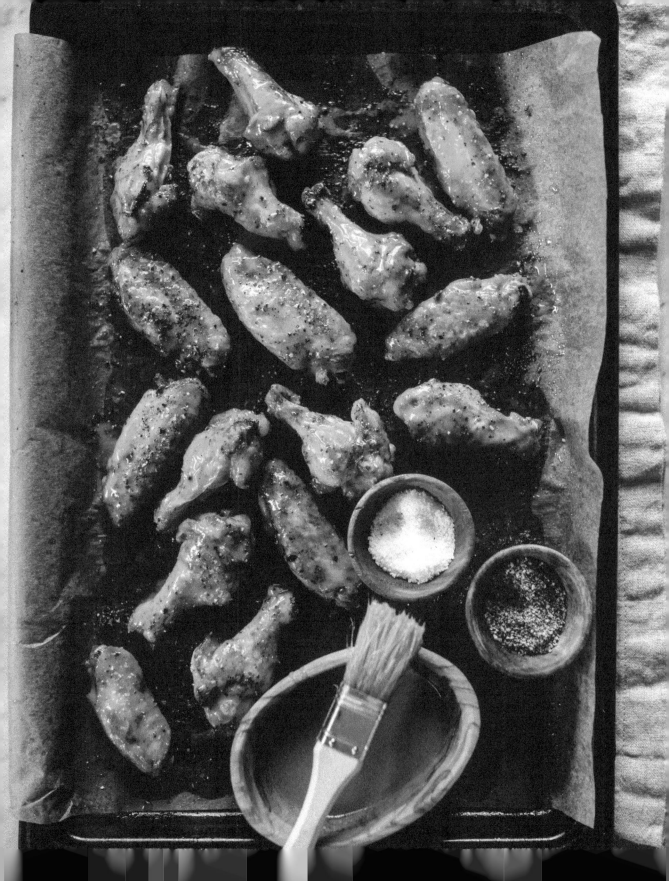

CHAPTER TWO

Setting Yourself Up for Success

Like so many things in life, good nutrition begins by planning ahead. Knowing which foods are best to have on hand, and also understanding how they fit together as complete, macronutrient-balanced meals are key to success. No matter how determined you may be, if you are overly hungry but without supplies or a plan, making the best decision for your nutrition needs becomes very difficult in the moment. The foods and pantry staples listed in this chapter will help set you up for stress-free success in achieving your goals.

What to Eat and What to Avoid

In order to achieve and maintain nutritional ketosis, the amount of carbohydrate at each meal must be kept exceptionally low, which means excluding foods that derive the majority of their energy (calories) from carbohydrates.

The obvious offenders are sweets, breads, pastas, and cereals, but even healthy foods such as many fruits, starchy vegetables, and whole grains contain carbohydrate levels that are too high to be included in most ketogenic meal plans. At the same time, just focusing on high-fat animal proteins as the staple of your meal plan can lead to protein ratios that are too high to support ketosis (see "Planning Your Macros," page 17), and potentially lead to increased inflammation and poor fat balance. In short, the balance of your macros and the quality of your food are both important.

The following table describes which foods should comprise the bulk of your diet, which can be included in moderation, and which should be avoided on a ketogenic diet.

Foods to Eat and Avoid on Keto

	FOODS TO ENJOY REGULARLY	FOODS TO EAT IN MODERATION	FOODS TO AVOID
VEGETABLES	Asparagus Celery Cruciferous vegetables (such as broccoli, cauliflower, Brussels sprouts) Eggplant Fennel Garlic Green beans Leafy greens (such as spinach, arugula, kale, radicchio lettuces) Mushrooms Onions Pickles Radishes Summer squash (zucchini and yellow squash)	Bell peppers (¼ cup serving) Carrots (¼ cup serving) Pumpkin and other winter squash (½ cup serving) Tomatoes (¼ cup serving)	Corn Peas Potatoes Yams/sweet potatoes
FISH AND SEAFOOD	All, with an emphasis on high-fat, wild-caught fish such as salmon, tuna canned in olive oil, sardines, and anchovies		
MEATS AND PROTEINS	Free-range eggs Free-range poultry Grass-fed beef and lamb Pasture-raised pork	Nitrate-free cured meats (such as some deli meat, bacon, salami, all-beef hot dogs)	Nitrate-containing processed meats (such as some deli meats) Sausage and bacon containing sugar or other fillers

	FOODS TO ENJOY REGULARLY	FOODS TO EAT IN MODERATION	FOODS TO AVOID
DAIRY AND CHEESE	Full-fat cheeses Full-fat cream cheese Grass-fed butter Heavy cream Sour cream	Full-fat cottage cheese (⅓ cup serving) Whole-milk Greek or Icelandic yogurt (½ cup serving)	Milk Processed cheeses, such as low-fat or part-skim cheese and cream cheese Sweetened yogurts
GRAINS AND LEGUMES			All, including peanuts
FRUITS	Avocados Dark berries (such as blueberries, raspberries, blackberries, and strawberries; limit to ¼ cup serving) Lemon juice Lime juice	Oranges and clementines (½ orange or 1 small clementine)	Higher-sugar fruits (such as apples, pears, peaches, plums, cherries, and melon)
NUTS, SEEDS, AND FLOURS	All tree nuts and nut butters (such as coconuts, almonds, Brazil nuts, cashews, filberts/hazelnuts, macadamia nuts, pecans, pine nuts, and walnuts) Chia, flax, and hemp seeds Pumpkin seeds Sesame seeds and tahini (sesame seed paste)	Almond flour Coconut flour	White flour, whole-wheat flour, chickpea flour, and rice flour
FATS AND OILS	Avocado oil and avocado mayo Coconut oil and full-fat unsweetened coconut milk MCT oil Olive oil and olives		Processed vegetable oils (such as canola, corn, and soybean)

	FOODS TO ENJOY REGULARLY	FOODS TO EAT IN MODERATION	FOODS TO AVOID
SWEETENERS, SPICES, AND SEASONINGS	Herbs (fresh or dried) such as basil, rosemary, mint, and parsley Red wine and apple cider vinegar Stone-ground mustard Unsweetened hot sauce Unsweetened spices and blends such as cinnamon, chili powder, red pepper flakes, black pepper, and salt Vanilla extract Worcestershire sauce	Balsamic vinegar (1 tablespoon serving) Natural sugar-free sweetener (monk fruit, stevia)	Artificial sweeteners (Splenda, Sweet'N Low) Barbecue sauce Ketchup Seasoning blends that include sugar (such as cinnamon sugar blend) Sugar of any kind (honey, maple syrup, brown sugar, cane sugar, corn syrup, agave) Sugar alcohols (erythritol, sorbitol)

Planning Your Macros

You'll want to stick to the 70-20-10 macro goal discussed in chapter 1 (page 5), and when thinking about your macros each day, each meal is just as important as the overall daily goal. If you consistently save all your daily protein or carbs for one meal, the ratios will be heavily skewed in that meal, which may prevent ketosis, causing cravings to come back and weight loss to stall, and making maintaining a plan more challenging. However, you are not a robot, and not every meal or every day is going to add up to fit the ratios exactly—that's okay! Instead of getting caught up in the ratios and numbers, think about the bigger picture: eating nutrient-dense real foods in the right combinations to achieve optimal health. Fortunately, the meal plans and recipes that follow are designed around this optimal macronutrient ratio and require no tracking to be successful.

All the macro math can be overwhelming. I get it—it's why I designed these meal plans to help you stay on track without having to count all the time! But for those who love numbers, there are several online resources to calculate your individual macronutrient needs based on age, height, weight, and activity level. If you would like to have specific daily targets, I suggest using an app such as MyFitness-Pal or Cronometer, both of which have free versions. The meal plans and recipes that follow are designed around a 1,300 to 1,600 daily calorie goal, which for most people will result in weight loss without having to calculate macros or track foods. To adjust this up or down, you can change the serving size of each recipe based on your hunger level, progress, and individual lifestyle needs.

What's the Story with Net Carbs?

Depending on your familiarity with a ketogenic diet, you may have heard of net carbs (grams of total carbs minus grams of fiber and grams of sugar alcohols). I encourage all of my clients to look at *total* carbs, not net, when tracking their macros. Food companies have become savvy to the keto trend, and have tried to capitalize on it with processed products touting low "net carbs." However, these often contain levels of total carbs that are too high to promote ketosis or good health. Plus, they're often loaded with filler fibers and gut-disrupting sweeteners, while also having little nutritional value.

The overwhelming majority of carbohydrates in the ideal diet should come from real foods, such as nonstarchy vegetables, which contain fiber in addition to a host of vitamins and minerals that are essential to healthy metabolic function and overall cell function. I recommend avoiding all boxed "keto-friendly" commercial products, such as breads, wraps, cereals, bars, and cookies. Instead, explore the delicious, real-food recipes in the chapters that follow. Your body will quickly adjust in a positive way to this shift in eating—you'll feel and function so much better, and many of those processed foods won't even taste so good anymore!

Setting Up Your Kitchen

A well-stocked refrigerator, freezer, and pantry make meal prep and balanced eating so much easier! The following list is a great starting point. You'll find many of these staple ingredients in the recipes to come, as well as convenience items you'll want to have on hand to whip up quick, easy meals and snacks.

PANTRY ITEMS

» Avocados: Store unripe avocados in a dark place at room temperature, but once they start to ripen, move them to the refrigerator so they last longer
» Broth or stock: chicken, beef, and vegetable

- » Canned diced and pureed tomatoes and tomato paste, no sugar added
- » Canned seafood, such as tuna packed in oil
- » Dried herbs such as dill, rosemary, parsley, and thyme
- » Nut and seed butters: unsweetened, such as almond, sunflower, and tahini (sesame seed paste)
- » Oils: Olive oil, avocado oil, coconut oil, and sesame oil
- » Spices: cinnamon, ground ginger, garlic powder, chili powder, ground cumin, and red pepper flakes
- » Vinegars: Red and white wine, unseasoned rice vinegar, and balsamic vinegar

REFRIGERATOR ITEMS

- » Butter, preferably grass-fed
- » Cheeses: Parmesan, cheddar, mozzarella, feta, goat cheese, and unflavored full-fat cream cheese
- » Cottage cheese, full-fat
- » Eggs, preferably free-range for the best quality fats
- » Greek yogurt, whole-milk
- » Mayonnaise
- » Salad greens: arugula, spinach, kale, baby lettuces, romaine, and mixed greens
- » Veggies, fresh: cucumber, bell pepper, cherry tomatoes, celery, broccoli, cauliflower, radishes, and carrots

FREEZER ITEMS

- » Frozen berries: strawberries, blueberries, raspberries, and blackberries
- » Frozen vegetables: broccoli, spinach/greens, green beans, asparagus, Brussels sprouts, bell peppers, cauliflower, riced cauliflower, zucchini, and yellow squash (avoid vegetable blends containing peas, corn, beans, or potatoes)
- » Meats, fish, and poultry
- » Nuts: almonds, walnuts, pecans, macadamia, hazelnuts, brazil nuts, and pistachios (store in the freezer to stay fresh longer!)
- » Seeds: flaxseed, chia seeds, pumpkin seeds, and sesame seeds

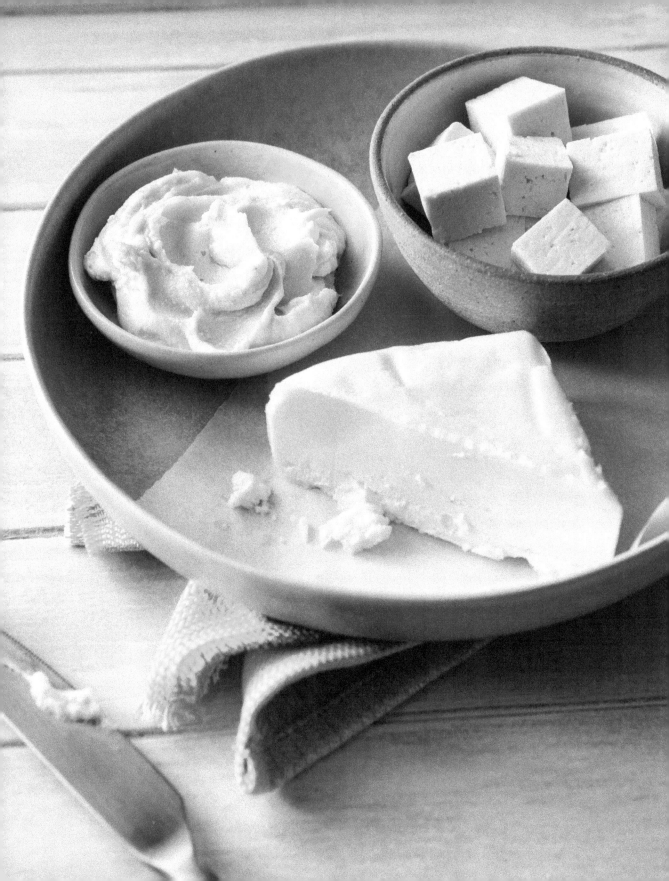

CHAPTER THREE

Meal Plans for Your First Four Weeks

Now that you understand the basic principles of a ketogenic lifestyle and realize how this way of eating can drastically improve your health and quality of life, it's time to start putting it all into practice!

One of the biggest challenges of sustaining a healthy keto diet is learning how to incorporate enough healthy fats into each meal to keep ratios in check without overdoing carbohydrates or protein levels. The 28-day meal plan provided in this chapter fits the ideal macronutrient ratios for a quick transition into ketosis and successful maintenance of that metabolic state. It's also geared specifically to the nutritional needs of those over 50 and allows for a wide variety of flavors and foods to keep things interesting.

For those who don't need as much variety in their day-to-day, you may choose to double up on some of the breakfast and lunch options and repeat favorites to cut down on cooking time. Do whatever works best for you to make your new lifestyle sustainable for your needs.

How to Use These Meal Plans to Create a Sustainable Diet

We all know that quick fixes and crash diets are never a good answer. Lifestyle and dietary changes are only effective when they are sustainable and long term. The foods must be enjoyable, the preparation realistic, and you shouldn't feel hungry or deprived! The meal plans and recipes in this book are designed to create that perfect balance of health, enjoyment, feasibility, and results. The specific weekly meal plans take all the guesswork out of meal prep so you know how to maintain a delicious ketogenic lifestyle, and the recipes and tips that follow allow for creative combinations to fit any palate or schedule.

Many of the recipes in this book have higher yields and can be prepped ahead to use throughout the week, freeing up time during busier weeks. I have marked these larger-yield recipes with an asterisk in the meal plans. Additionally, the weekly plans assume each recipe will feed two people, so if you are cooking for just one, you may choose to use leftovers more frequently to cut down on the amount of cooking. Alternatively, note which options are freezer-friendly and work ahead to stock your freezer with made-ahead delicious meals for additional weeks!

You'll find a shopping list for each week with all the fresh ingredients you'll need. The weeks do build on each other, and the pantry lists and many of the canned goods and refrigerated condiments will be used again in future weeks, so it is important to start with Week 1 if you are relying on the shopping lists.

These meal plans all include three meals a day, with the option of a snack as needed. They all fall within a daily caloric range of 1,400 to 1,600 calories, and hit the ideal ketogenic ratios of 70 to 75 percent fat, 15 to 20 percent protein, and 5 to 10 percent carbohydrates. You may see some initial weight loss when transitioning into ketosis, but this range should allow for maintenance of a healthy weight.

For those with a goal of weight loss, transitioning to only two meals each day after the first one to two weeks, or omitting snacks entirely, may help achieve this goal (see "What You Should Know About Intermittent Fasting," page 23, and "The Lowdown on Snacks," page 27). This will keep calories at 1,200 to 1,400 calories daily, while maintaining ideal ketogenic ratios. These calorie ranges may be higher or lower than what you are used to aiming for with either weight loss or weight maintenance goals, but often what we eat matters more than simply focusing on how much we eat. Plus, when adhering to strict ketogenic dietary ratios, most people find they are not as hungry as they were previously and that they are able to achieve weight goals without counting or reducing overall calories.

What You Should Know About Intermittent Fasting

Intermittent fasting, or time-restricted eating, can help deepen your level of ketosis as well as aid with weight loss if that's your goal. When your body must rely on stored body fat as an energy source between meals, rather than dietary fat from meals or snacks, it increases brain-boosting ketone production for energy in the absence of any other fuel source, and also draws from stored energy (body fat), which can lead to sustainable and healthy weight loss.

The goal of shortening the "window of eating" is not to decrease overall caloric intake, although this may happen naturally for some people, but just to shorten the time frame in which you ingest that energy. Implementing intermittent fasting should be a gradual progression, and never forced. Most of my clients find that after the first two or three weeks of a ketogenic diet, they naturally have increased satiety and many transition comfortably to a longer "fasting" window between their last meal and first meal of the following day.

If you wish to transition to a longer fasting window, try pushing breakfast back 30 minutes every two to three days so that after a few weeks, you have gradually increased the time between dinner and breakfast the following day to 16 to 18 hours (such as a 6:00 or 7:00 p.m. dinner and a 10:00 or 11:00 a.m. breakfast/brunch), giving your body more time to work on burning stored energy and deepening ketosis.

For many, a 6-hour eating window/18-hour fasting schedule means only two larger meals each day; others prefer to stick with three meals within that eating window. Again, this should feel natural and never forced, so do what is most comfortable for you. It is important to maintain adequate protein intake, especially as we age, so I do not advise transitioning to only one meal a day for long periods of time. I've designed the weekly meal plans that follow to include more "snack" breakfast options, as you may find your hunger for breakfast decreases, you desire something lighter, or prefer to move this meal option to more of a snack between the first and third meal of the day.

WEEK 1

	MONDAY	TUESDAY	WEDNESDAY	
MEAL 1	Zucchini-Nut Muffin (page 52) *(freeze ⅔ of batch for future weeks)**	Pimento Cheese Scrambled Eggs (page 56) *(make Bacon-Studded Pimento Cheese* [page 75] ahead for week)*	Leftover Zucchini-Nut Muffins	
MEAL 2	Keto Waldorf Chicken Salad* (page 64) with celery sticks	Leftover Keto Waldorf Chicken Salad on ½ slice Microwave Keto Bread (page 120)	Leftover Cheesy Southwestern Meat Loaf with 2 cups mixed greens with 2 tablespoons leftover Red Wine Vinaigrette (page 128)	
MEAL 3	Cheesy Southwestern Meat Loaf* (page 102) with 2 cups mixed greens with 2 tablespoons Red Wine Vinaigrette* (page 128)	Slow Cooker White Chicken Chili* (page 94) *(freeze ½ recipe for week 3)* with 1 cup cooked kale or spinach sautéed in 1 tablespoon olive oil	Parchment-Baked Cod and Asparagus with Beurre Blanc* (page 86)	
DAILY NUTRITION	**Macronutrients:** 77% Fat, 19% Protein, 4% Carbs **Per day:** Calories: 1238; Total Fat: 106g; Saturated Fat: 26g; Protein: 58g; Total Carbs: 13g; Fiber: 5g; Net Carbs: 8g	**Macronutrients:** 75% Fat, 19% Protein, 6% Carbs **Per day:** Calories: 1340; Total Fat: 112g; Saturated Fat: 38g; Protein: 65g; Total Carbs: 18g; Fiber: 6g; Net Carbs: 12g	**Macronutrients:** 77% Fat, 19% Protein, 4% Carbs **Per day:** Calories: 1191; Total Fat: 102g; Saturated Fat: 41g; Protein: 57g; Total Carbs: 13g; Fiber: 4g; Net Carbs: 8g	

	THURSDAY	FRIDAY	SATURDAY	SUNDAY
	Yogurt Parfait with Creamy Blueberry Crumble* (page 50)	Pimento Cheese Scrambled Eggs (page 56) *(with leftover Bacon-Studded Pimento Cheese)*	Cheesy Cauliflower Grits* (page 53) topped with 2 eggs fried in 1 tablespoon olive oil	Leftover Yogurt Parfait with Creamy Blueberry Crumble
	Leftover Bacon-Studded Pimento Cheese sandwich on Microwave Keto Bread (page 120)	Taco salad made with crumbled leftover Cheesy Southwestern Meat Loaf, 2 cups mixed greens, and 2 tablespoons ranch dressing *(no sugar added)*	½ cup cottage cheese with ¼ cup berries, 2 tablespoons nuts, and 1 tablespoon melted coconut oil *(no recipe required!)*	Leftover Cheesy Cauliflower Grits topped with 1/2 portion leftover Shrimp Scampi with Zucchini Noodles
	Leftover Slow Cooker White Chicken Chili with 2 cups mixed greens with 2 tablespoons leftover Red Wine Vinaigrette	Leftover Parchment-Baked Cod and Asparagus with Beurre Blanc*	Shrimp Scampi with Zucchini Noodles* (page 85)	Baked Spaghetti Squash Carbonara with Chicken* (page 96)
	Macronutrients: 78% Fat, 13% Protein, 9% Carbs **Per day:** Calories: 1463; Total Fat: 127g; Saturated Fat: 46g; Protein: 47g; Total Carbs: 33g; Fiber: 11g; Net Carbs: 22g	**Macronutrients:** 78% Fat, 16% Protein, 6% Carbs **Per day:** Calories: 1779; Total Fat: 155g; Saturated Fat: 55g; Protein: 73g; Total Carbs: 23g; Fiber: 10g; Net Carbs: 13g	**Macronutrients:** 76% Fat, 18% Protein, 6% Carbs **Per day:** Calories: 1307; Total Fat: 111g; Saturated Fat: 44g; Protein: 58g; Total Carbs: 20g; Fiber: 5g; Net Carbs: 15g	**Macronutrients:** 76% Fat, 14% Protein, 10% Carbs **Per day:** Calories: 1591; Total Fat: 135g; Saturated Fat: 57g; Protein: 56g; Total Carbs: 36g; Fiber: 8g; Net Carbs: 28g

Keto Flu

Many people experience symptoms of "keto flu," or clinical dehydration, when trying a ketogenic diet for the first time. Symptoms include nausea, fatigue, headache, and light-headedness, usually start three to four days in, and can last anywhere from one to two weeks. This phenomenon is due to the quick dumping of stored water as the body breaks down glycogen stores within the first few days of a very low carbohydrate diet. This is a normal side effect of this metabolic process and not specific to age, gender, or specific medical conditions. While uncomfortable, it is not cause for alarm. More importantly, keto flu can be avoided entirely by following these two tips:

Stay hydrated. Water will be your best friend in fighting keto flu. As a general rule, I suggest drinking half of your body weight in ounces of water each day. So, if you weigh 200 pounds, aim for 100 ounces of water a day. This can come in the form of unsweetened teas, seltzers, or water infused with berries or a slice of grapefruit or orange.

Keep up with your electrolytes. The main four electrolytes are sodium, potassium, calcium, and magnesium. While there are many electrolyte supplement drinks out there, many also have added sugars, so try to get these essentials through your diet. Avocados are high in potassium and magnesium. Nuts, seeds, and fatty fish such as salmon and tuna packed in oil are good sources of magnesium. You can also drink some chicken or beef broth, which is high in sodium, to boost electrolytes. However, if you are on a medically supervised low-sodium diet, consult with your doctor before increasing sodium levels.

The Lowdown on Snacks

Here are a handful of ideas for quick and easy healthy snacks should you find yourself in need of a little something extra. Typically, snacks are helpful during the first week, as your body has not fully transitioned into ketosis and may continue to crave carbs or sugars. However, cravings are reduced and hunger is diminished as your body relies more on stored body fat for energy between meals. Especially if weight loss is a goal, or you just want to achieve a deeper level of ketosis for increased energy and mental clarity, I suggest avoiding snacks after the first one to two weeks.

→ ¼ cup cottage cheese and ¼ cup fresh berries

→ 2 sliced strawberries with 2 tablespoons heavy cream, whipped to ¼ cup

→ 1 tablespoon almond butter or peanut butter with celery sticks

→ ½ avocado mashed with 1 ounce tuna or leftover chicken, or
   1 hard-boiled egg

→ Cucumber slices with 2 tablespoons cream cheese and 10 capers or 5 olives

→ 1 ounce cubed feta marinated in olive oil

→ 1 Pecan Sandy Fat Bomb (page 78)

→ ¼ cup Cashew Hummus (page 122) and green bell pepper slices

Week 1 Shopping List

PRODUCE

- Apple, Granny Smith (1 small)
- Asparagus (8 ounces)
- Avocados (3)
- Cauliflower (1 small head or 2 cups fresh riced)
- Celery (1 bunch)
- Cilantro (1 bunch)
- Garlic (1 head)
- Kale or spinach (2 cups)
- Lemons (3)
- Limes (2)
- Mixed greens (12 ounces)
- Onion, red (1 small)
- Onion, yellow (1 small)
- Parsley, Italian (1 bunch)
- Scallions (1 bunch)
- Spinach, baby (2 cups)
- Squash, spaghetti (1 small)
- Zucchini (5 large)

SEAFOOD, POULTRY, AND MEAT

- Bacon (10 ounces)
- Chicken thighs, boneless, skinless (5 pounds)
- Fish, fresh white flaky, such as cod or halibut, skinned (1 pound)
- Ground beef, preferably grass-fed (1 pound)
- Ground pork chorizo or spicy Italian sausage (1 pound)
- Shrimp, peeled and deveined (1 pound)

DAIRY AND EGGS

- Butter, unsalted, preferably grass-fed (3 sticks)
- Cheese, cheddar, shredded (2¾ cups)
- Cheese, cottage, full-fat (1 cup)
- Cheese, cream (24 ounces)
- Cheese, Mexican, shredded (2 cups)
- Cheese, Parmesan, shredded (2¼ cups)
- Eggs, large, preferably free-range (14)
- Heavy cream (2 cups)
- Sour cream (½ cup)
- Yogurt, plain full-fat Greek (2 cups)

FROZEN ITEMS

- ❑ Blueberries (1¼ cups)

CANNED AND BOTTLED ITEMS

- ❑ Chicken bone broth, 2 cups
- ❑ Chiles, diced mild green, 2 (4-ounce) cans
- ❑ Chipotle in adobo (1 can)
- ❑ Dressing, ranch (no sugar added)
- ❑ Pimentos, jarred diced drained (4 ounces)
- ❑ Tomato paste, no sugar added, 1 (6-ounce) can
- ❑ White wine, dry

PANTRY ITEMS

(Items with an asterisk will also be needed for future weeks and will not be included on those shopping lists. Also restock things like olive oil and almond flour as needed.)

- ❑ Almond flour*
- ❑ Almonds, slivered (¼ cup)
- ❑ Baking powder*
- ❑ Baking soda*
- ❑ Cinnamon, ground*
- ❑ Coriander, ground*
- ❑ Cumin, ground*
- ❑ Flaxseed/flax meal, ground*
- ❑ Garlic powder*
- ❑ Ginger, ground*
- ❑ Granulated sugar-free sweetener (monk fruit, stevia, etc.)*
- ❑ Mayonnaise*
- ❑ Mustard, Dijon*
- ❑ Oil, olive*
- ❑ Onion powder*
- ❑ Oregano, dried
- ❑ Pepper, ground*
- ❑ Red pepper flakes*
- ❑ Salt*
- ❑ Tarragon, dried*
- ❑ Vanilla extract*
- ❑ Vinegar, red wine and white wine*
- ❑ Walnuts or roasted unsalted pecans (1½ cups)

TIP: Vitamin D and calcium go hand in hand to promote bone health as we age. Wonderful dietary sources of both of these important micronutrients include yogurt made with whole milk and oily canned fish, such as salmon, tuna, mackerel, and sardines, which often include small edible bones that are loaded with calcium. You can swap out any of the lunch recipes for canned fish on a simple mixed greens salad paired with 2 tablespoons of nuts or seeds and half an avocado for a quick and easy meal that is full of powerful nutrition.

WEEK 2

	MONDAY	TUESDAY	WEDNESDAY	
MEAL 1	Leftover Zucchini Nut-Muffin *(frozen from week 1)*	Keto Peanut Butter Cup* (page 124) *(make ahead and freeze for later weeks)*	The Best Deviled Eggs* (page 68)	
MEAL 2	Leftover Baked Spaghetti Squash Carbonara with Chicken *(from week 1)*	Cream of Tomato Soup* (page 65) with grilled cheese made with Microwave Keto Bread (page 120) and 1 ounce cheese	Leftover Weeknight Chili	
MEAL 3	Weeknight Chili* (page 108)	Leftover Baked Spaghetti Squash Carbonara with Chicken *(from week 1)* with 1 cup chopped romaine with 1 tablespoon Easiest Creamy Caesar Dressing* (page 129)	Baked Buffalo Chicken Wings* (page 89) with Garlicky Creamed Spinach* (page 72)	
DAILY NUTRITION	**Macronutrients:** 74% Fat, 16% Protein, 10% Carbs **Per day:** Calories: 1360; Total Fat: 112g; Saturated Fat: 32g; Protein: 56g; Total Carbs: 32g; Fiber: 11g; Net Carbs: 21g	**Macronutrients:** 79% Fat, 13% Protein, 8% Carbs **Per day:** Calories: 1534; Total Fat: 135g; Saturated Fat: 46g; Protein: 49g; Total Carbs: 30g; Fiber: 7g; Net Carbs: 23g	**Macronutrients:** 76% Fat, 16% Protein, 8% Carbs **Per day:** Calories: 1520; Total Fat: 128g; Saturated Fat: 38g; Protein: 61g; Total Carbs: 31g; Fiber: 13g; Net Carbs: 18g	

	THURSDAY	FRIDAY	SATURDAY	SUNDAY
	Leftover Zucchini-Nut Muffin *(frozen from week 1)*	2 eggs scrambled in 1 tablespoon of olive oil or butter	Bagels and Lox* (page 62)	Omelet with 2 eggs, 1 ounce cheese, ¼ cup mushrooms, and ½ cup chopped spinach sautéed in 2 tablespoons olive oil
	Leftover Baked Buffalo Chicken Wings with 1 cup chopped romaine and 1 tablespoon leftover Easiest Creamy Caesar Dressing (page 129)	Leftover Cream of Tomato Soup with leftover Deviled Eggs	1/2 portion leftover Baked Buffalo Chicken Wings	1/2 portion leftover Bagels and Lox
	Leftover Weeknight Chili over ½ cup cauliflower rice	Leftover Baked Buffalo Chicken Wings with leftover Garlicky Creamed Spinach	Crispy Baked Pork Chops with Mushroom Gravy (page 116)	Leftover Crispy Baked Pork Chops with Mushroom Gravy tossed with 2 cups zoodles
	Macronutrients: 75% Fat, 17% Protein, 8% Carbs **Per day:** Calories: 1282; Total Fat: 107g; Saturated Fat: 29g; Protein: 53g; Total Carbs: 27g; Fiber: 11g; Net Carbs: 16g	**Macronutrients:** 80% Fat, 13% Protein, 7% Carbs **Per day:** Calories: 1560; Total Fat: 138g; Saturated Fat: 53g; Protein: 52g; Total Carbs: 23g; Fiber: 7g; Net Carbs: 16g	**Macronutrients:** 76% Fat, 18% Protein, 6% Carbs **Per day:** Calories: 1600; Total Fat: 135g; Saturated Fat: 46g; Protein: 73g; Total Carbs: 23g; Fiber: 9g; Net Carbs: 14g	**Macronutrients:** 76% Fat, 17% Protein, 7% Carbs **Per day:** Calories: 1661; Total Fat: 140g; Saturated Fat: 46g; Protein: 72g; Total Carbs: 25g; Fiber: 11g; Net Carbs: 14g

Week 2 Shopping List

PRODUCE

- Avocados (3)
- Basil, fresh (1 cup)
- Bell pepper, green (1)
- Cauliflower (½ cup riced)
- Garlic (2)
- Lemon (1)
- Lettuce, romaine (4 ounces)
- Mushrooms (6 ounces)
- Onions, yellow (3 small)
- Onion, red (1 small)
- Parsley, Italian (1 bunch)
- Rosemary, fresh (1 bunch)
- Spinach (½ cup chopped)
- Tomatoes, medium (4)
- Zucchini (1 large)

SEAFOOD, POULTRY, AND MEAT

- Chicken wings (4 pounds)
- Ground beef, preferably grass-fed (1 pound)
- Ground Italian sausage, mild or spicy (8 ounces)
- Pork, boneless chops (1 pound)
- Salmon, smoked (6 ounces)

DAIRY AND EGGS

- Butter, unsalted, preferably grass-fed (2 sticks)
- Cheese, cream (20 ounces)
- Cheese, cheddar or other, shredded (4 ounces)
- Cheese, mozzarella, shredded (2½ cups)
- Cheese, Parmesan, freshly grated (½ cup)
- Eggs, large, preferably free-range (12)
- Heavy cream (2 cups)
- Sour cream (1 cup)

FROZEN ITEMS

- Spinach (1 pound)

CANNED AND BOTTLED ITEMS

☐ Capers
☐ Olives, green pitted

☐ Tomatoes, diced,
1 (14½-ounce) can
☐ Tomato paste, 1 (6-ounce) can

PANTRY ITEMS

(Items with an asterisk will also be needed for future weeks and are not included on those shopping lists. Keep an eye on things like olive oil, mayonnaise, and almond flour, as you may need to restock.)

☐ Anchovy paste
☐ Cacao butter (½ cup)
☐ Cocoa powder,
unsweetened (¼ cup)
☐ Chili powder
☐ Dressing, blue cheese
☐ Hot sauce (such as Tabasco or
Frank's RedHot)
☐ Paprika, smoked

☐ Peanut butter or almond butter,
unsweetened creamy*
☐ Sage, dried
☐ Seeds, chia or whole flaxseed
☐ Seeds, poppy
☐ Seeds, sesame*
☐ Stock, chicken (3 cups)
☐ Thyme, dried
☐ Walnuts (¼ cup)
☐ Worcestershire sauce*

TIP: Some people find that their bowel patterns shift as they transition to a ketogenic diet. This isn't necessarily specific to keto, but rather a side effect of your body adjusting to different foods. A properly formulated ketogenic diet should provide all the dietary fiber needed to maintain healthy digestive function, but be sure to not skimp on natural fiber-dense foods such as green leafy vegetables, cruciferous vegetables like cabbage and cauliflower, nuts, seeds, berries, and avocados. And remember to hydrate, hydrate, hydrate! Water is the best natural detoxifier and system lubricant that we have.

WEEK 3

	MONDAY	TUESDAY	WEDNESDAY	
MEAL 1	1/2 portion leftover Bagels and Lox (from week 2)	Leftover Zucchini-Nut Muffin (frozen from week 1)	2 eggs scrambled in 1 tablespoon of olive oil topped with 2 tablespoons Any-Herb Pesto* (page 123)	
MEAL 2	Leftover Slow Cooker White Chicken Chili (frozen from week 1)	2 cups mixed greens, 4 ounces leftover steak, 2 tablespoons leftover Easiest Creamy Caesar Dressing (from week 2), ½ avocado	Leftover Cauliflower Fried Rice Bowl with a fried egg and ½ avocado	
MEAL 3	Steak with Blue Cheese Butter* (page 110) and 1 cup green beans sautéed in 1 tablespoon olive oil	Stir-Fried Chicken and Broccoli with Cashews* (page 90) with Cauliflower Fried Rice* (page 121)	Coconut-Crusted Salmon with Avocado Sauce* (page 88)	
DAILY NUTRITION	**Macronutrients:** 74% Fat, 19% Protein, 7% Carbs **Per day:** Calories: 1452; Total Fat: 120g; Saturated Fat: 44g; Protein: 68g; Total Carbs: 24g; Fiber: 9g; Net Carbs: 15g	**Macronutrients:** 73% Fat, 21% Protein, 6% Carbs **Per day:** Calories: 1362; Total Fat: 110g; Saturated Fat: 41g; Protein: 70g; Total Carbs: 23g; Fiber: 8g; Net Carbs: 15g	**Macronutrients:** 77% Fat, 15% Protein, 8% Carbs **Per day:** Calories: 1525; Total Fat: 130g; Saturated Fat: 44g; Protein: 58g; Total Carbs: 28g; Fiber: 16g; Net Carbs: 12g	

	THURSDAY	FRIDAY	SATURDAY	SUNDAY
	Leftover Keto Peanut Butter Cup *(frozen from week 2)*	Crunchy Granola Bars (page 77) *(freeze for snacks and week 4)*	2 eggs scrambled in 2 tablespoons leftover Any-Herb Pesto	Leftover Keto Peanut Butter Cup *(frozen from week 2)*
	2 cups zoodles tossed with 2 tablespoons leftover Any-Herb Pesto and 4-ounce can tuna packed in olive oil	Roasted Greek Cauliflower* (page 69) topped with a fried egg	Egg Roll in a Bowl (page 60)	1/2 portion leftover Roasted Greek Cauliflower with 4 ounces pulled rotisserie chicken
	Leftover Slow Cooker White Chicken Chili *(frozen from week 1)*	Leftover Coconut-Crusted Salmon with Avocado Sauce	Leftover Roasted Greek Cauliflower with 4 ounces pulled rotisserie chicken	Slow Cooker Swedish Meatballs* (page 114) with 2 cups zoodles
	Macronutrients: 70% Fat, 22% Protein, 8% Carbs **Per day:** Calories: 1249; Total Fat: 97g; Saturated Fat: 30g; Protein: 70g; Total Carbs: 24g; Fiber: 8g; Net Carbs: 16g	**Macronutrients:** 76% Fat, 15% Protein, 9% Carbs **Per day:** Calories: 1215; Total Fat: 103g; Saturated Fat: 44g; Protein: 47g; Total Carbs: 25g; Fiber: 13g; Net Carbs: 12g	**Macronutrients:** 75% Fat, 18% Protein, 7% Carbs **Per day:** Calories: 1910; Total Fat: 160g; Saturated Fat: 44g; Protein: 88g; Total Carbs: 28g; Fiber: 8g; Net Carbs: 20g	**Macronutrients:** 69% Fat, 24% Protein, 7% Carbs **Per day:** Calories: 1105; Total Fat: 85g; Saturated Fat: 37g; Protein: 66g; Total Carbs: 18g; Fiber: 5g; Net Carbs: 13g

Week 3 Shopping List

PRODUCE

(Items with an asterisk will be used in week 4.)

- Arugula (4 ounces)
- Avocados (2)
- Basil, fresh (1 cup)
- Bell pepper, red (1)
- Broccoli crowns (2 cups)
- Cabbage, napa or savoy (1 head)*
- Cauliflower, small (2 heads)
- Celery (1 bunch)
- Garlic (1 head)
- Ginger, 1 (3-inch) piece*
- Green beans (2 cups)
- Lemon (1)
- Limes (2)
- Mixed greens (8 ounces)
- Onion, yellow (2)
- Parsley, Italian (1 bunch)
- Scallions (1 bunch)*
- Spinach, baby (2 cups)
- Zucchini (3 large)

SEAFOOD, POULTRY, AND MEAT

- Beef, filet mignon or New York strip, 4 (4-ounce) steaks
- Chicken, boneless, skinless thighs (1 pound)
- Chicken, cooked rotisserie (1)
- Ground beef, preferably grass-fed (1 pound)
- Ground pork sausage (1½ pounds)
- Salmon, 4 skinless fillets (1 pound total)

DAIRY AND EGGS

- Eggs, large, preferably free-range (12)
- Butter, unsalted, preferably grass-fed (¼ cup)
- Cheese, blue, crumbled (¼ cup)
- Cheese, cream (4 ounces)
- Cheese, feta (8 ounces)
- Cheese, goat (4 ounces)
- Cheese, Parmesan, shredded (½ cup)
- Heavy cream (1½ cups)
- Sour cream (1 cup)

CANNED AND BOTTLED ITEMS

- Olives, Kalamata, pitted (1 jar)

PANTRY ITEMS

(Items with an asterisk will also be needed for future weeks and are not included on those shopping lists.)

- ☐ Allspice, ground
- ☐ Almond butter, unsweetened
- ☐ Almonds, slivered (1 cup)
- ☐ Cashews, whole unsalted
- ☐ Coconut milk, full-fat
- ☐ Coconut, unsweetened flaked
- ☐ Flour, coconut
- ☐ Oil, coconut*
- ☐ Oil, sesame*
- ☐ Pecans, roasted unsalted (1 cup)

- ☐ Pumpkin seeds, shelled (1 cup)
- ☐ Soy sauce*
- ☐ sriracha or other hot sauce
- ☐ Stock, beef (1½ cups)
- ☐ Tahini
- ☐ Tuna, packed in olive oil, 2 (4-ounce) cans
- ☐ Vinegar, rice wine*
- ☐ Walnuts (1 cup)

TIP: If you suffer from hot flashes, you'll want to hear this: Regular dietary intake of soy isoflavones (a compound found in many plants) from foods like tofu, tempeh, and edamame has been shown to reduce instance and severity of hot flashes in menopausal women. Fortunately, tofu is a low-carb protein option and a keto-friendly way to increase soy consumption. Try replacing the chicken in Tuesday's stir-fry with cubed or crumbled tofu, and scramble some tofu in place of the eggs with Saturday's breakfast.

WEEK 4

	MONDAY	TUESDAY	WEDNESDAY	
MEAL 1	Leftover Zucchini-Nut Muffin *(frozen from week 1)*	Leftover Keto Peanut Butter Cup *(frozen from week 2)*	2 eggs scrambled with ¼ cup Spinach and Artichoke Dip* (page 76)	
MEAL 2	Leftover Slow Cooker Swedish Meatballs	Leftover Cheesy Chicken and Broccoli Casserole	Leftover Slow Cooker Swedish Meatballs with frozen cauliflower rice	
MEAL 3	Cheesy Chicken and Broccoli Casserole* (page 91)	Leftover Slow Cooker Swedish Meatballs on a Microwave Keto Bread (page 120) sandwich	Leftover Cheesy Chicken and Broccoli Casserole	
DAILY NUTRITION	**Macronutrients:** 80% Fat, 16% Protein, 4% Carbs **Per day:** Calories: 1378; Total Fat: 122g; Saturated Fat: 49g; Protein: 54g; Total Carbs: 16g; Fiber: 5g; Net Carbs: 11g	**Macronutrients:** 80% Fat, 15% Protein, 5% Carbs **Per day:** Calories: 1581; Total Fat: 141g; Saturated Fat: 56g; Protein: 60g; Total Carbs: 18g; Fiber: 6g; Net Carbs: 12g	**Macronutrients:** 79% Fat, 16% Protein, 5% Carbs **Per day:** Calories: 1648; Total Fat: 144g; Saturated Fat: 59g; Protein: 67g; Total Carbs: 21g; Fiber: 7g; Net Carbs: 14g	

	THURSDAY	FRIDAY	SATURDAY	SUNDAY
	Leftover Crunchy Granola Bar *(from week 3)*	2 eggs scrambled with ¼ cup leftover Spinach and Artichoke Dip	Leftover Crunchy Granola Bar *(from week 3)*	Leftover Biscuits and Gravy
	Egg Roll in a Bowl (page 60)	Leftover Brussels Sprouts with Pancetta and Walnuts	Biscuits and Gravy* (page 58)	Leftover Keto Peanut Butter Cup *(frozen from week 2)*
	Brussels Sprouts with Pancetta and Walnuts* (page 70) topped with a fried egg	Slow Cooker Herb-and-Garlic Short Rib Stew (page 109)	Leftover Slow Cooker Herb-and-Garlic Short Rib Stew	Clam Chowder (page 84) with 2 cups mixed greens with 1 tablespoon leftover Easiest Creamy Caesar Dressing *(from week 2)*
	Macronutrients: 78% Fat, 13% Protein, 9% Carbs **Per day:** Calories: 1467; Total Fat: 127g; Saturated Fat: 19g; Protein: 47g; Total Carbs: 34g; Fiber: 12g; Net Carbs: 22g	**Macronutrients:** 76% Fat, 14% Protein, 10% Carbs **Per day:** Calories: 1451; Total Fat: 123g; Saturated Fat: 33g; Protein: 52g; Total Carbs: 34g; Fiber: 13g; Net Carbs: 21g	**Macronutrients:** 76% Fat, 16% Protein, 8% Carbs **Per day:** Calories: 1559; Total Fat: 131g; Saturated Fat: 46g; Protein: 62g; Total Carbs: 33g; Fiber: 12g; Net Carbs: 21g	**Macronutrients:** 76% Fat, 17% Protein, 7% Carbs **Per day:** Calories: 1664; Total Fat: 140g; Saturated Fat: 64g; Protein: 69g; Total Carbs: 31g; Fiber: 7g; Net Carbs: 24g

Week 4 Shopping List

PRODUCE

- ❑ Bell pepper, red (1)
- ❑ Broccoli florets (1 pound)
- ❑ Brussels sprouts (1 pound)
- ❑ Cabbage (2 cups finely chopped or 1 bag coleslaw mix)
- ❑ Carrot (1)
- ❑ Cauliflower, fresh (1 small head or 2 cups cut)
- ❑ Celery (1 bunch)
- ❑ Garlic (2 heads)
- ❑ Ginger
- ❑ Lime (1)
- ❑ Mixed greens (2 cups)
- ❑ Mushrooms (8 ounces)
- ❑ Onions, yellow (2)
- ❑ Parsley, Italian (1 bunch)

SEAFOOD, POULTRY, AND MEAT

- ❑ Bacon (4 ounces)
- ❑ Beef, short ribs, boneless (1 pound)
- ❑ Chicken, boneless, skinless thighs (1 pound)
- ❑ Clams, chopped, 3 (6½-ounce) cans
- ❑ Ground pork sausage (14 ounces)
- ❑ Pancetta (4 ounces)

DAIRY AND EGGS

- ❑ Butter, unsalted, preferably grass-fed (1 stick)
- ❑ Cheese, cheddar, shredded (2¾ cups)
- ❑ Cheese, goat (4 ounces)
- ❑ Cheese, mozzarella, shredded (½ cup)
- ❑ Cheese, Parmesan, shredded (¾ cup)
- ❑ Cream cheese (16 ounces)
- ❑ Eggs, large, preferably free-range (12)
- ❑ Heavy cream (2 cups)
- ❑ Sour cream (½ cup)

FROZEN ITEMS

- ❑ Cauliflower rice
- ❑ Spinach (8 ounces)

CANNED AND BOTTLED ITEMS

- Artichoke hearts, 1 (14-ounce) can
- Clam juice, bottled (8 ounces)
- Stock, beef (3 cups)
- Stock, vegetable (1 cup)
- Wine, Merlot or Cabernet Sauvignon

PANTRY ITEMS

- Almonds, slivered (¼ cup)
- Bone broth, chicken or beef (½ cup)
- Tomatoes, diced, 1 (14½-ounce) can
- Vinegar, balsamic
- Walnuts (½ cup)

TIP: By this week you may find yourself feeling less hungry for the full three meals a day, or maybe just moving breakfast back a bit later. I've made the breakfast options in this week a bit lighter and more "snack-like" to accommodate this natural progression. If you're interested in and ready to practice intermittent fasting, this week's schedule provides a great platform for that. You may want to hold off on breakfast, start your day with meal 2, and save the meal 1 food for a midday snack. Or, if you'd like to move to two meals a day, simply skip the breakfast suggestion entirely and enjoy meals 2 and 3 in an 8- to 10-hour window. Do what feels natural and comfortable for your body and hunger levels.

Tips for Continuing Past Four Weeks

As you use the recipes and meal plans in this book, you will learn how to build your own healthy ketogenic plate with the correct ratios of macronutrients. You'll also start to feel more comfortable in social or dining-out situations. This is such an important part of making this a sustainable lifestyle! These tips for building your own meal plan will give you the confidence to get creative.

Match proteins to fats. Generally, to keep ratios optimal for ketosis, make sure to include 1 tablespoon of healthy fats (olive oil, butter, mayonnaise, avocado, nuts/seeds) for every ounce of protein such as fish, meat, and poultry, or every 1 egg. For example, if you're eating a 4-ounce piece of salmon, you could sauté this in 1 tablespoon of olive oil, top with 2 tablespoons of pesto or aioli, and serve with sliced avocado.

Make veggies a vehicle for getting in more fat. Think of all your colorful nonstarchy vegetables, such as salad greens, broccoli, cauliflower, asparagus, green beans, eggplant, etc. as a super nutritious way to get the healthy fats you need into each meal. Drizzling a tablespoon or two of olive oil onto a salad or sautéed veggies is a great way to keep the fat ratios of each meal keto-friendly.

Flavor your fats. Pestos and aiolis are condiments to use to get a variety of flavors into your fats. An aioli is a thinner version of mayonnaise that contains added flavor from garlic and other herbs or spices. You can buy these premade or whip up a simple version by adding roasted garlic and lemon juice to basic mayonnaise. Pestos, or herbs blended with olive oil, nuts, and garlic, are delicious with meats, fish, eggs, or sautéed vegetables. Try making your own Any-Herb Pesto (page 123) or use a store-bought version for convenience.

Don't eat when you're not hungry. This may seem like a no-brainer, but eating just because it's mealtime or out of boredom is never a healthy practice. Similarly, skipping meals when you are hungry can lead to negative health consequences. Listen to your body. If it is telling you it needs fuel, maybe you need to push mealtime earlier, or fit in a snack during your day. If you're still full from lunch, maybe you don't need a full dinner that night. One of the benefits of a ketogenic diet is that all those satiating, nutrient-dense foods you're eating prevent constant cravings for empty filler foods, and most people find they eat less of higher quality foods, as well.

Dining out is okay, too. Most restaurants now offer low-carb or keto-friendly options, but carbs and sugars can be hidden in sauces and dressings. Your best bet is to order a protein along with nonstarchy vegetables or a side salad. You can add healthy fats such as unsweetened dressings (like ranch, blue cheese, or oil and vinegar), guacamole, a drizzle of olive oil, or extra butter.

Don't arrive to a restaurant or party hungry! It can be hard to resist the chips, breads, and other carb-heavy fillers if you haven't eaten all day. One or two hours before dining out, enjoy a snack with healthy fats, such as a Pecan Sandy Fat Bomb (page 78) or Crunchy Granola Bar (page 77), to help keep a handle on hunger and cravings.

SIMPLE AND QUICK MEALS

While I love creating and enjoying a wide variety of crowd-pleasing recipes, I stress to my patients the importance of knowing that not every meal has to be an elaborate recipe. A good repertoire of simple and quick "recipe-less" meals will help you sustain healthy dietary changes even during the busiest of times. Some of my favorites include:

Oven-Roasted Vegetables: Roasting makes any veggie tastier, and the hands-off cooking time (no sautéing!) is a huge plus. Cut the veggies to a uniform size so they cook evenly, toss with plenty of olive oil, salt, pepper, and other herbs or spices, and roast at 425°F on a foil-lined baking sheet until crispy and cooked to desired doneness. Of course, the bigger the veggie, the longer the roasting time. Broccoli, cauliflower, Brussels sprouts, green beans, and asparagus are all delicious roasted.

Slow-Cooked Meats with Jarred Sauces: Beef, chicken, and pork all cook up beautifully in the slow cooker, and with a jarred sauce you don't have to do a thing but dump in and push go! Chicken thighs and jarred pesto with a splash of broth or cream is a favorite in my house, but you could try pork and Italian dressing, beef and blue cheese dressing with a splash of broth, or chicken and (no sugar added) salsa. Shred the cooked meat and serve with zoodles, atop a salad, or with roasted veggies.

Brinner (breakfast for dinner): Eggs don't have to be reserved for the morning! A simple omelet cooked in butter or oil, made with fresh or frozen spinach or other veggies and drizzled with olive oil or pesto, or topped with avocado or guacamole, contains the perfect keto-friendly balance of macros and is on the table in under 10 minutes.

Kitchen Sink Salad: Top mixed greens with whatever leftover proteins you have at the end of the week—chicken, fish, beef, pork, hard-boiled eggs, or canned fish. Add a variety of healthy fats such as nuts, seeds, avocado, and olives, and don't forget a big drizzle of olive oil to top it off.

Freezer Clean-Out Stir-Fry: Frozen veggies work best in a stir-fry, and I always keep several bags on hand for busy nights. Broccoli, peppers, green beans, and asparagus are some of my favorites. Fry them up in olive oil with whatever protein you have on hand, flavor with soy sauce, sesame oil, and some hot sauce, then serve topped with chopped nuts or seeds.

MAKE LEFTOVERS

No one wants to be a short-order cook, stuck making a new meal (or several different meals!) every day. Eating leftovers is the best way to cut down on frequent cooking, but not everyone loves eating the same dish several times. I recommend embracing the "one protein, many meals" concept. Make a big batch of roasted chicken or meat and repurpose it for many different meals. Meal 1 can be chicken and roasted veggies, meal 2 could be a chicken salad with mayo and avocado, meal 3 could be chicken tossed with zoodles and jarred pesto, and meal 4 could be a chicken Cobb salad.

About the Recipes

I've included nutrition-focused labels on the recipes that follow to highlight the power of the real-food ingredients included in each meal. Food is the best medicine we have, and every meal we enjoy has the power to improve our health and well-being. Look for the following labels throughout the recipe chapters:

Reduces Inflammation. These recipes include anti-inflammatory ingredients like omega-3 fatty acid–rich fish, avocados, nuts, seeds, and herbs and spices.

Bone Health. These recipes have ingredients with higher calcium, like dark leafy greens, yogurt, and some cheeses, or that include good sources of vitamin D like eggs and fatty fish, to help your body better absorb dietary calcium.

Protein Power. These recipes are complete protein meals to sustain muscle mass and metabolic function.

Freezer-Friendly. These recipes have a higher yield or can be doubled and frozen for later use.

Brain Health. These recipes include brain-boosting ingredients like fish and eggs, as well as higher fat ratios for greater ketone production and sustained energy and mental clarity.

PART TWO

THE RECIPES

Preparing healthy, delicious, keto-friendly meals at home shouldn't feel like a full-time job, and not every meal has to be a complicated recipe. The recipes that follow are designed for the novice cook and require minimal special ingredients outside of the staples listed in the previous section. I believe that the best tasting and most satiating food is simple food, and that means sticking to real ingredients; adding natural flavor from herbs, spices, and aromatics such as garlic and citrus zest; and whenever possible, eating what is fresh and in season. The following recipes contain a wide variety of spices, but minimal use of added sweeteners. Sugar substitutes are okay to use in dessert recipes when you have a hankering for something sweet, but these foods are best thought of as "treats" rather than staples in your day-to-day diet. A ketogenic lifestyle doesn't mean finding "keto alternatives" for all of your carb-heavy favorites, but rather adopting and embracing a new way of eating, full of new flavors, foods, and combinations!

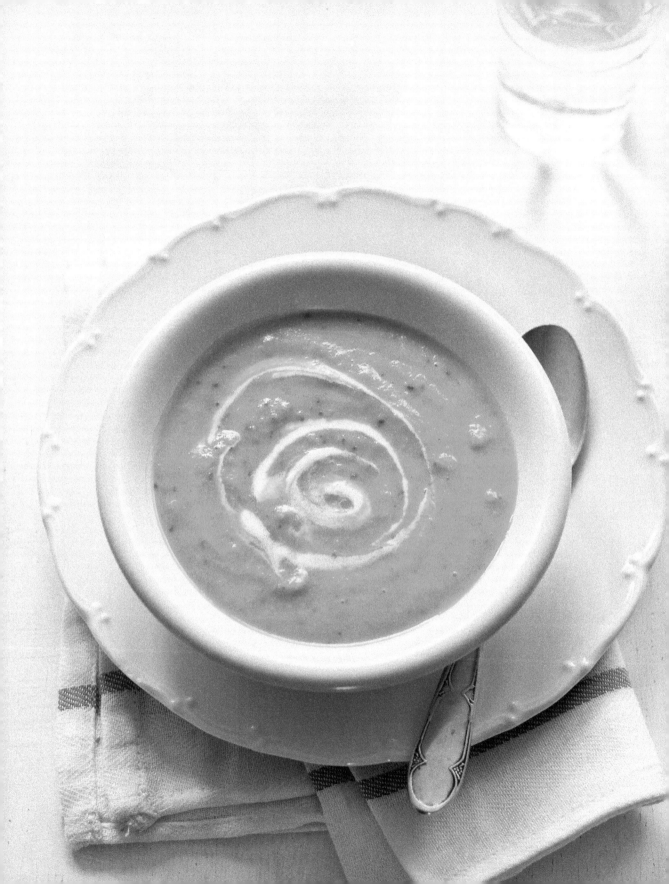

CHAPTER FOUR

Breakfast & Midday Meals

Yogurt Parfait with Creamy Blueberry Crumble

SERVES 4

Prep Time: 10 minutes, plus 10 minutes to rest

Cook Time: 25 minutes

Protein Power

Plain Greek yogurt is a convenient source of protein, but not everyone enjoys the flavor or texture. This recipe is a great way to make it fun and tasty. Any berry, or even a mix of several, such as raspberry, blackberry, and strawberry, would be delicious in this dish. I tend to default to frozen berries, as they are available year-round and are perfect for a last-minute dish. Feel free to use fresh berries if you prefer.

6 tablespoons cold unsalted butter, divided

¼ cup almond flour

¼ cup ground flaxseed

¼ cup slivered almonds

¼ cup chopped roasted unsalted walnuts

1 cup fresh or frozen blueberries

2 to 4 tablespoons granulated sugar-free sweetener

Zest of 1 lemon

1 teaspoon vanilla extract

½ teaspoon ground ginger or cinnamon

½ cup heavy cream

2 cups plain full-fat Greek yogurt

1. Preheat the oven to 350°F and generously coat the bottom and sides of an 8-inch square glass baking dish or 8-inch pie pan with 2 tablespoons of butter.

2. In a medium bowl, cut the remaining 4 tablespoons of butter into very small pieces. Add the almond flour, flaxseed, almonds, and walnuts and mix until crumbly. Set aside.

3. In a separate bowl, combine the blueberries, sweetener, lemon zest, vanilla extract, and ginger or cinnamon. Toss to coat the blueberries well.

4. Add the blueberry mixture to the prepared baking dish (they won't quite cover the bottom), and pour the heavy cream over the blueberry mixture.

5. Top the blueberry mixture evenly with the flour-and-nut mixture, and bake for 20 to 25 minutes, until golden brown. Let rest for 10 minutes before serving to allow the mixture to thicken.

6. To serve, top one-quarter of the warm crumble mixture with ½ cup of Greek yogurt.

MAKE-AHEAD TIP: Prepare the crumble over the weekend and have it on hand for a quick and easy breakfast all week. For an added bonus, double the crumble recipe and serve warm with fresh whipped cream as a special dessert. Leftover crumble can be stored covered in the refrigerator for up to 4 days.

MACRONUTRIENTS: 79% Fat, 8% Protein, 13% Carbs

PER SERVING: Calories: 500; Total Fat: 45g; Saturated Fat: 22g; Protein: 10g; Total Carbs: 18g; Fiber: 5g; Net Carbs: 13g

Zucchini-Nut Muffins

MAKES 12

Prep Time: 15 minutes / **Cook Time:** 20 minutes

Reduces Inflammation

While you'll find many keto baked good recipes on the Internet, few have much nutritional value and they end up just being extra calories. This can inhibit you from reaching your goals—and to boot, they often don't even taste good. These muffins, conversely, are filled with anti-inflammatory properties from flaxseed, olive oil, ground cinnamon, ginger, and nuts. Using olive oil in baked goods may seem odd, but it's a common practice in the Mediterranean region, and it adds a buttery flavor to this delicious heart-healthy treat.

Butter or coconut oil, for greasing (optional)

1½ cups shredded zucchini (1 large or 2 small zucchini)

1 teaspoon salt

2 large eggs

⅓ cup granulated sugar-free sweetener of choice (monk fruit, stevia, etc.)

¼ cup extra-virgin olive oil (or melted coconut oil)

1¾ cups almond flour

¼ cup ground flaxseed or flax meal

1 teaspoon baking soda

½ teaspoon ground cinnamon

½ teaspoon ground ginger (optional)

½ cup chopped walnuts or pecans, plus 2 tablespoons finely chopped nuts

1. Preheat the oven to 350°F. Line a 12-muffin tin with liners or coat well with butter or coconut oil.

2. Drain the zucchini: Place the shredded zucchini in a colander or on several layers of paper towels. Sprinkle with the salt and let sit for 10 minutes. Using another paper towel, press on the zucchini to release any excess moisture.

3. In a large bowl, whisk together the eggs, granulated sweetener, and olive oil. Add the zucchini, almond flour, flaxseed, baking soda, cinnamon, and ginger and mix until well incorporated. Stir in ½ cup of chopped nuts.

4. Divide the batter evenly between the 12 prepared muffin cups, filling each about three-quarters full. Sprinkle 2 tablespoons of finely chopped nuts evenly among the 12 filled muffin tins. Bake until a toothpick inserted in the center of a muffin comes out clean, 15 to 18 minutes.

VARIATION TIP: I love using citrus zest such as lemon, orange, or grapefruit in my baked goods to increase flavor and allow for less sweetener. I suggest adding 1 to 2 tablespoons of zest, or to taste.

MACRONUTRIENTS: 79% Fat, 11% Protein, 10% Carbs

PER SERVING: Calories: 170; Total Fat: 16g; Saturated Fat: 2g; Protein: 5g; Total Carbs: 4g; Fiber: 2g; Net Carbs: 2g

Cheesy Cauliflower Grits

SERVES 4

Prep Time: 5 minutes / **Cook Time:** 15 minutes

Bone Health

Much like Cream of Wheat in the North, grits are a quick and easy staple as part of a larger breakfast spread in the South. Incredibly versatile, they can be paired with a breakfast protein such as sausage, bacon, or a fried egg for a complete meal, or serve as the base for a hearty comfort dish when topped with sautéed shrimp, fish, or pulled pork or chicken. Traditional grits are made from corn, which is mostly carbohydrate and not a part of a ketogenic diet. This version uses riced cauliflower for a low-carb, high-fiber, keto-friendly treat. Is there anything cauliflower can't do?

¼ cup heavy cream

4 tablespoons unsalted butter, divided

1 teaspoon salt

½ teaspoon garlic powder

¼ teaspoon freshly ground black pepper

2 cups riced cauliflower (see ingredient tip)

¾ cup shredded cheddar cheese

¼ cup shredded Parmesan cheese

1. In a medium saucepan over high heat, combine the heavy cream, 2 tablespoons of butter, salt, garlic powder, and pepper and bring to just below a boil. Add the riced cauliflower and reduce heat to low.

2. Simmer, stirring occasionally, for 8 to 10 minutes, until the cauliflower is tender, most of the water from the vegetable has evaporated, and the mixture is thick and creamy.

3. Remove from the heat and stir in the shredded cheeses and remaining 2 tablespoons of butter. Serve warm.

INGREDIENT TIP: Fresh riced cauliflower works best in this recipe for texture and consistency, but you can use prepared frozen riced cauliflower if you prefer. If using frozen, increase cooking time by 3 to 4 minutes to ensure all the excess moisture has been released. To prepare fresh, separate the florets from the core of half a head of cauliflower and place in the bowl of a food processor. Pulse until the cauliflower resembles small grains of rice or couscous. Alternatively, you can finely shred the florets using a large box grater. Reserve the remaining cauliflower for another use.

MACRONUTRIENTS: 82% Fat, 12% Protein, 6% Carbs

PER SERVING: Calories: 280; Total Fat: 26g; Saturated Fat: 16g; Protein: 8g; Total Carbs: 5g; Fiber: 1g; Net Carbs: 4g

Cheesy Keto Hash Browns with Avocado Mayo

SERVES 4
Prep Time: 15 minutes / **Cook Time:** 20 minutes

Reduces Inflammation

Topped with a creamy avocado mayo and filled with protein from almond flour and ground flaxseed, these hash browns are a great complete vegetarian breakfast or midday meal. For extra protein, top with a fried egg. This dish is high in heart-healthy omega-3 fatty acids from the flaxseed, olive oil, and avocado, and loaded with vitamin E from the almond flour, making it an anti-inflammatory powerhouse. Cooked hash browns will freeze nicely for up to 3 months; to maintain their crispy texture, place frozen hash browns on a baking sheet lined with foil and greased with oil, and reheat in a preheated 400°F oven until heated through, 5 to 8 minutes.

2 cups riced cauliflower, fresh or frozen

2 ounces cream cheese, room temperature

2 tablespoons ground flaxseed or flax meal

2 tablespoons almond flour

½ teaspoon garlic powder

1 teaspoon baking powder

1 teaspoon salt, divided

1 large egg, lightly beaten

2 tablespoons minced scallions, green and white parts

6 tablespoons extra-virgin olive oil, divided

1 small very ripe avocado, peeled, pitted, and mashed

1 teaspoon white wine vinegar or lemon juice

¼ teaspoon freshly ground black pepper

1. Steam or microwave the riced cauliflower, covered, until tender. For frozen, cook 2 to 3 minutes in the microwave or 4 to 5 minutes on the stovetop. For fresh, cook 1 to 2 minutes in the microwave or 3 to 4 minutes on the stovetop. Set aside until completely cooled.

2. Meanwhile, in a medium bowl, mix the cream cheese until smooth. Add the flaxseed, almond flour, garlic powder, baking powder, ½ teaspoon of salt, and the beaten egg and whisk to combine well.

3. When the cauliflower reaches room temperature, cover with a paper towel. Use your hands to press down, allowing the liquid to rise above the towel, and pour off the excess. Continue pressing until the cauliflower is mostly dried and drained of excess liquid.

4. Stir the cauliflower and scallions into the cream cheese mixture.

5. Heat 2 tablespoons of olive oil in a large skillet over medium heat. Drop heaping tablespoonfuls of the cauliflower batter onto the skillet, and press down with a spatula to form 4 to 6 small patties, depending on the size of the skillet. Cook for 2 to 4 minutes, until the bottom is browned, then flip and cook another 2 to 4 minutes. Repeat with another 2 tablespoons of olive oil and the remaining batter.

6. To prepare the avocado mayo, in a small bowl, blend the remaining 2 tablespoons of olive oil, the mashed avocado, the remaining ½ teaspoon of salt, the vinegar or lemon juice, and pepper and whisk or beat with a fork until smooth and creamy.

7. Serve the hash browns warm with avocado mayo.

VARIATION TIP: You can use shredded zucchini in place of the riced cauliflower in this recipe. Drain the excess water off first by placing the shredded zucchini in a colander or on several layers of paper towels. Sprinkle with ½ teaspoon of salt and let sit for 10 minutes. Using another layer of paper towels, press down on the zucchini to release any excess moisture and pat dry.

MACRONUTRIENTS: 85% Fat, 6% Protein, 9% Carbs

PER SERVING: Calories: 379; Total Fat: 37g; Saturated Fat: 7g; Protein: 6g; Total Carbs: 10g; Fiber: 6g; Net Carbs: 4g

Pimento Cheese Scrambled Eggs

SERVES 2

Prep Time: 2 minutes / **Cook Time:** 3 minutes

Protein Power

The cooking technique of low heat and constant stirring produces the creamiest scrambled eggs, and the addition of pimento cheese keeps the fat ratios high and makes a tasty alternative to boring everyday eggs. Make a large batch of Bacon-Studded Pimento Cheese (page 75) to have on hand throughout the week for snacks and recipes such as this one.

4 large eggs

½ teaspoon salt

¼ teaspoon freshly ground black pepper

2 tablespoons unsalted butter

¼ cup Bacon-Studded Pimento Cheese (page 75)

1. In a small bowl, whisk together the eggs, salt, and pepper. Set aside.

2. Melt the butter in a small skillet over medium heat. Add the whisked eggs and reduce heat to low. Stirring constantly with a spatula, scramble the eggs for 1 to 2 minutes, until no longer runny, but not fully cooked through.

3. Remove the skillet from the heat and stir in the pimento cheese for an additional 30 seconds, or until melted and well combined.

INGREDIENT TIP: You can substitute store-bought pimento cheese or 3 tablespoons of shredded cheddar cheese mixed with 1 tablespoon of mayonnaise if you don't have any on hand.

MACRONUTRIENTS: 79% Fat, 19% Protein, 2% Carbs

PER SERVING: Calories: 353; Total Fat: 31g; Saturated Fat: 14g; Protein: 17g; Total Carbs: 2g; Fiber: 0g; Net Carbs: 2g

Cream Chipped Beef with Arugula

SERVES 2

Prep Time: 5 minutes / **Cook Time:** 10 minutes

Protein Power

This open-faced sandwich is a true comfort dish that brings back memories of my childhood. My mom made this the traditional way with canned dried beef and no veggies in sight, but this version uses leftover cooked steak (or deli roast beef). The addition of wilted arugula makes it significantly lower in sodium and higher in micronutrients, and some dried herbs give it a richer flavor.

2 tablespoons unsalted butter

1 tablespoon almond flour

1 ounce cream cheese, room temperature

½ teaspoon dried thyme or other herb such as rosemary, oregano, or sage

¼ teaspoon freshly ground black pepper

½ cup heavy cream

8 ounces cooked steak, cut into very thin strips, or deli roast beef (see ingredient tip)

2 cups baby arugula (or chopped fresh baby spinach leaves)

1 Microwave Keto Bread round (page 120), halved and toasted

1. Melt the butter in a medium saucepan over low heat. Add the almond flour and whisk for 1 minute, until slightly browned. Add the cream cheese, thyme, and pepper, and whisk until the cheese is melted, 1 to 2 minutes.

2. Increase heat to medium-high. Whisking constantly, stream in the cream and continue whisking until thickened, 3 to 4 minutes. Add the sliced steak and arugula, reduce heat to low, and stir to combine. Cook for another 1 to 2 minutes, or until the beef is heated through and the arugula is wilted.

3. To serve, top each toasted sandwich round half with half of the beef and arugula mixture.

INGREDIENT TIP: Using leftover cooked steak helps this dish come together in a flash. You can substitute 8 ounces of thinly sliced deli roast beef, which is lowest in sodium of all deli meats, in place of the steak if you prefer. Simply slice the roast beef into thin strips and add to the sauce just as you would the steak.

MACRONUTRIENTS: 76% Fat, 22% Protein, 2% Carbs

PER SERVING: Calories: 703; Total Fat: 59g; Saturated Fat: 30g; Protein: 38g; Total Carbs: 5g; Fiber: 1g; Net Carbs: 4g

Biscuits and Gravy

SERVES 4

Prep Time: 20 minutes / **Cook Time:** 20 minutes

This cozy protein-rich dish is perfect for a weekend brunch or midday larger meal. Using bone broth instead of chicken stock or broth adds extra collagen-rich protein, which is great for skin, joint, and gut health, as well as helping to reduce the signs of aging. You can substitute ground turkey or chicken for the pork sausage if you prefer; just choose dark meat rather than lean to keep the fat-to-protein ratios in check.

For the biscuits

1 cup almond flour

1½ teaspoons baking powder

½ teaspoon salt

2 tablespoons cold unsalted butter, diced

2 tablespoons heavy cream

½ cup shredded mozzarella or cheddar cheese

1 large egg

For the gravy

8 ounces ground Italian pork sausage (not sweet)

4 ounces cream cheese, room temperature

½ cup heavy cream

½ cup chicken or beef bone broth

1 teaspoon onion powder

1 teaspoon salt

¼ teaspoon freshly ground black pepper

1. **To make the biscuits.** Preheat the oven to 375°F and line a large baking sheet with parchment paper.

2. In a large bowl, combine the almond flour, baking powder, and salt and mix well. Add the butter, and use a fork to crumble into the flour mixture until it resembles coarse pebbles.

3. Use the fork to whisk in the heavy cream, 1 tablespoon at a time. Whisk in the cheese and egg until a smooth dough forms.

4. Cut the dough into four equal pieces and form each into a ball. Place on the prepared baking sheet, pressing down slightly with the heel of your palm to flatten a bit, and bake for 16 to 18 minutes, or until golden brown.

5. **To make the gravy.** While the biscuits bake, brown the sausage in a medium saucepan over medium heat until cooked through, 3 to 4 minutes. Do not drain the rendered fat.

6. Add the cream cheese, heavy cream, bone broth, onion powder, salt, and pepper to the sausage and reduce heat to low. Stirring constantly, simmer until thickened, another 6 to 8 minutes.

7. Halve the biscuits horizontally and serve topped with gravy.

MAKE-AHEAD TIP: If you want to make a larger batch of biscuit dough to have on hand throughout the week, store the formed dough covered in the refrigerator for 2 to 3 days, or wrapped tightly and frozen for up to 3 months. Extra biscuit dough can be used in the Biscuit-Topped Chicken Pot Pie (page 92).

MACRONUTRIENTS: 82% Fat, 12% Protein, 6% Carbs

PER SERVING: Calories: 674; Total Fat: 63g; Saturated Fat: 27g; Protein: 20g; Total Carbs: 9g; Fiber: 3g; Net Carbs: 6g

Egg Roll in a Bowl

SERVES 2

Prep Time: 10 minutes / **Cook Time:** 10 minutes

Reduces Inflammation

This fun dish has all the flavor of a takeout favorite without the hidden carbs and sugars. This is a filling, easy-to-prepare meal that will soon become a favorite. Feel free to mix up the nonstarchy veggies or swap out the proteins—this bowl would be equally delicious with shrimp or pulled chicken. The spicy mayo is an excellent garnish for other meats or even with raw veggies for a snack. It keeps well in the refrigerator for up for two weeks, so make extra and enjoy it for several meals!

2 large eggs

2 tablespoons sesame oil, divided

2 tablespoons soy sauce, divided

2 tablespoons extra-virgin olive oil

6 ounces ground pork

1 tablespoon chopped fresh ginger (or 1 teaspoon ground ginger)

2 cloves garlic, minced

2 cups finely chopped cabbage (or bagged coleslaw mix; no dressing)

2 ribs celery, diced

½ small red bell pepper, diced

2 tablespoons lime juice, divided

2 scallions, minced (green and white parts)

2 tablespoons mayonnaise

1 teaspoon sriracha or other hot sauce

½ teaspoon garlic powder

1. In a small bowl, beat together the eggs, 1 tablespoon of sesame oil, and 1 tablespoon of soy sauce and set aside.

2. Heat the olive oil in a large skillet over medium heat. Sauté the ground pork, breaking it apart, until browned and no longer pink, 4 to 5 minutes. Add the ginger and garlic and sauté for an additional 30 seconds.

3. Add the cabbage, celery, and bell pepper and sauté, stirring constantly, until the vegetables are wilted and fragrant, another 2 to 3 minutes.

4. Push the vegetables and pork to one side of the skillet and add the egg mixture to the other side. Reduce heat to low and scramble the egg until cooked through, 1 to 2 minutes. Remove the skillet from the heat and mix the egg into the pork and cabbage.

5. In a small bowl, whisk together the remaining 1 tablespoon of sesame oil, the remaining 1 tablespoon of soy sauce, 1 tablespoon of lime juice, and the scallions. Pour over the cooked pork mixture and stir to combine well, reserving the bowl.

6. In the same small bowl, combine the remaining 1 tablespoon of lime juice, the mayonnaise, sriracha, and garlic powder.

7. Divide the pork mixture evenly between two bowls and drizzle each with half of the spicy mayo. Serve warm.

INGREDIENT TIP: I like napa or savoy cabbage for their tenderness and slightly sweet flavor. If you use green or red cabbage, you may need to sauté it slightly longer for it to cook down.

MACRONUTRIENTS: 78% Fat, 14% Protein, 8% Carbs

PER SERVING: Calories: 695; Total Fat: 61g; Saturated Fat: 14g; Protein: 25g; Total Carbs: 14g; Fiber: 4g; Net Carbs: 10g

Bagels and Lox

SERVES 6

Prep Time: 10 minutes / **Cook Time:** 20 minutes

Protein Power

This brunch favorite doesn't have to be off-limits on a ketogenic diet! This variation uses an adapted "fathead" dough. While this dough is low-carb, it is not ketogenic on its own due to the high ratio of protein to fat. I add high-healthy fats in the form of smoked salmon and olive oil to round out the macros, and limit the portion size to half a bagel. Store leftover bagels in the freezer for this dish or a quick and easy breakfast of a bagel slathered with almond or peanut butter.

8 ounces cream cheese, room temperature, divided

2½ cups shredded mozzarella or Swiss cheese (not cheddar)

1½ cups almond flour

1 tablespoon baking powder

2 large eggs, beaten

1 tablespoon sesame seeds

1 tablespoon poppy seeds

1 tablespoon whole flaxseed or chia seeds

¼ cup extra-virgin olive oil

2 tablespoons chopped capers (optional)

6 ounces smoked salmon

2 tablespoons very thinly sliced red onion

1. Preheat the oven to 400°F and line a baking sheet with parchment paper.

2. Place 2 ounces of cream cheese in a medium microwave-safe bowl and mash well with a fork. Add the shredded cheese and stir to combine. Microwave on high for 1½ minutes, or until the cheeses start to melt. Stir well and microwave on high for an additional 30 to 90 seconds, or until well melted and smooth when stirred.

3. While the cheese melts, combine the almond flour and baking powder in a large bowl, breaking up any lumps. Whisk in the beaten eggs.

4. Add the melted cheese mixture to the almond flour mixture and knead the dough with your hands for 3 to 4 minutes or until the cheese is well incorporated into the flour. The dough will be very sticky.

5. In a small bowl, mix together the sesame seeds, poppy seeds, and flaxseed. Set aside.

6. Divide the dough into six even balls and roll each out to a 6-inch log. Curve the log to form a circle, pressing the ends together to seal. Dip the front of each bagel into the bowl of seeds, pressing so they stick. Place each bagel 4 inches apart on the prepared baking sheet.

7. Bake for 12 to 15 minutes, or until golden brown. Remove from the oven, transfer to a cooling rack, and allow to cool to the touch.

8. To assemble the lox, slice three bagels in half (reserving the other three for another use). In a small bowl, combine the remaining 6 tablespoons of cream cheese, the olive oil, and capers (if using) and whisk until smooth.

9. Top each bagel half with 2 tablespoons of cream cheese mixture, 1 ounce of smoked salmon, and a few slivered red onions.

VARIATION TIP: These bagels are also delicious topped with a sliced avocado, a fried egg, and a drizzle of olive oil and seasonings to round out the macros and make a complete meal.

MACRONUTRIENTS: 74% Fat, 18% Protein, 8% Carbs

PER SERVING: Calories: 575; Total Fat: 49g; Saturated Fat: 16g; Protein: 26g; Total Carbs: 11g; Fiber: 4g; Net Carbs: 7g

Keto Waldorf Chicken Salad

SERVES 4

Prep Time: 5 minutes

Brain Health

Next time you roast or grill a batch of chicken thighs, make some extra to use in this simple and quick salad. It's a huge time-saver for midweek lunches or a hearty snack. With the perfect blend of proteins and fat, and just the right amount of apple for flavor and crunch, this salad has it all and supports brain-boosting ketone production. Serve atop a bed of mixed greens, in a lettuce wrap, as a sandwich using Microwave Keto Bread (page 120), or on its own straight out of the bowl!

½ cup mayonnaise

1 tablespoon Dijon mustard

1 teaspoon salt

½ to 1 teaspoon dried tarragon or other herb such as rosemary, oregano, or thyme (optional)

¼ teaspoon freshly ground black pepper

2 cups chopped cooked chicken thighs (or pulled rotisserie chicken)

2 ribs celery, chopped

½ small Granny Smith apple, cored and seeded, diced

½ cup chopped walnuts or pecans

1. In a medium bowl, combine the mayonnaise, mustard, salt, tarragon (if using), and pepper.

2. Add the chopped chicken to the mayonnaise mixture. Add the celery, apple, and walnuts and stir to combine well.

3. Store leftovers covered in the refrigerator for up to 3 days.

MACRONUTRIENTS: 76% Fat, 20% Protein, 4% Carbs

PER SERVING: Calories: 435; Total Fat: 37g; Saturated Fat: 6g; Protein: 20g; Total Carbs: 5g; Fiber: 2g; Net Carbs: 3g

Cream of Tomato Soup

SERVES 4
Prep Time: 10 minutes, plus 10 minutes to cool
Cook Time: 40 minutes

Freezer-Friendly

This rich and creamy tomato soup is slightly higher in carbohydrate ratios on its own, but if you round it out with a higher fat and protein salad, such as the Keto Waldorf Chicken Salad (page 64), or pair it with a grilled cheese sandwich made with Microwave Keto Bread (page 120), it's a perfect, complete ketogenic meal. This soup freezes well, so consider making a larger batch when tomatoes are in season and freezing it in one- or two-serving portions to have on hand when you need a comfort meal!

4 medium whole tomatoes, cored

8 medium garlic cloves, peeled

½ medium yellow onion, quartered

¼ cup extra-virgin olive oil, divided

2 tablespoons fresh rosemary (or 2 teaspoons dried)

1 teaspoon salt, plus more

1 cup chicken or vegetable stock

1 cup heavy cream, divided

1 cup fresh basil, roughly chopped

1 tablespoon balsamic or red wine vinegar

¼ to ½ teaspoon red pepper flakes

1. Preheat the oven to 400°F.

2. In a bowl, combine the tomatoes, garlic cloves, onion quarters, 2 tablespoons of olive oil, the rosemary, and salt. Toss to coat the vegetables with the oil. Transfer to an 8-inch square glass baking dish, cover with aluminum foil, and roast until the tomatoes have released most of their juices, 30 to 35 minutes. Allow to cool for 10 minutes.

3. Transfer the contents of the baking dish, including the liquids, to a blender, or transfer to a large bowl and use an immersion or stick blender. Add the stock, the remaining 2 tablespoons of olive oil, ¾ cup of the cream, the basil, vinegar, and red pepper flakes and blend until smooth and creamy.

4. Transfer the mixture to a medium saucepan and heat over medium-low heat, stirring constantly, until heated through. Season to taste with additional salt if desired and serve warm, drizzled with the remaining cream.

INGREDIENT TIP: For added protein and nutrition, use bone broth in place of the stock. Bone broth is also a great source of collagen, which helps with skin, hair, nail, and gut health as we age.

MACRONUTRIENTS: 87% Fat, 3% Protein, 10% Carbs

PER SERVING: Calories: 364; Total Fat: 36g; Saturated Fat: 15g; Protein: 3g; Total Carbs: 10g; Fiber: 2g; Net Carbs: 8g

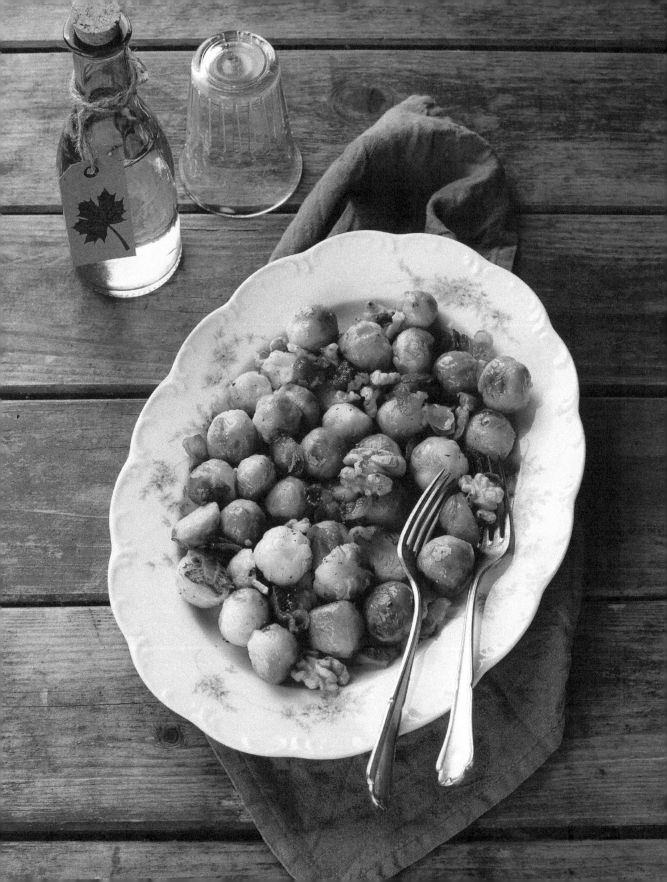

CHAPTER FIVE

Sides & Snacks

The Best Deviled Eggs

SERVES 4

Prep Time: 15 minutes, plus 30 minutes to chill

Protein Power

Deviled eggs are so simple to make, and having a batch in the refrigerator means you'll always have a protein-rich grab-and-go snack at the ready. This version uses omega-3-rich anchovy paste, olive oil, and olives for a unique flavor and added health bonus. If you're serving these for a crowd, you can make them look fancier by placing the filling into a piping bag and making a design when you fill the eggs, but for a faster method, simply spooning the filling in will do the trick!

1 tablespoon mayonnaise

1 tablespoon extra-virgin olive oil

1 teaspoon Dijon mustard

1 teaspoon anchovy paste

¼ teaspoon freshly ground black pepper

4 large hard-boiled eggs, shelled

8 pitted green olives, chopped

1 tablespoon red onion, minced

1 tablespoon fresh parsley, minced

1. In a small bowl, whisk together the mayonnaise, olive oil, mustard, anchovy paste, and pepper. Set aside.

2. Slice the hard-boiled eggs in half lengthwise, remove the yolks, and place the yolks in a medium bowl. Reserve the egg white halves and set aside.

3. Smash the yolks well with a fork and stir in the mayonnaise mixture. Add the olives, onion, and parsley and stir to combine.

4. Spoon the filling into each egg white half. Cover and chill for 30 minutes or up to 24 hours before serving cold.

VARIATION TIP: You could make an egg salad with the same ingredients. Rather than halving the eggs, chop or grate each whole shelled egg on a box grater directly into the mayonnaise mixture and stir to combine well.

MACRONUTRIENTS: 76% Fat, 21% Protein, 3% Carbs

PER SERVING: Calories: 137; Total Fat: 12g; Saturated Fat: 3g; Protein: 7g; Total Carbs: 1g; Fiber: 0g; Net Carbs: 1g

Roasted Greek Cauliflower

SERVES 6

Prep Time: 10 minutes / **Cook Time:** 35 minutes

Bone Health

Rich, creamy, and full of wonderful flavor, this unique spin on roasted cauliflower will breathe new life into that old keto standby, cauliflower! I prefer the taste and texture of authentic Greek feta cheese, which is made from sheep's milk rather than cow's milk. It's worth seeking out if you can find it.

6 cups cauliflower florets (1 medium head cauliflower)

½ cup extra-virgin olive oil, divided

1 teaspoon dried oregano

½ teaspoon salt

¼ teaspoon freshly ground black pepper

10 pitted Kalamata olives, coarsely chopped

2 cups baby spinach leaves, coarsely chopped

¼ cup fresh parsley leaves, coarsely chopped

8 ounces crumbled feta cheese, divided

4 ounces goat cheese

½ cup heavy cream

1. Preheat the oven to 425°F.

2. In a large bowl, combine the cauliflower florets, ¼ cup of olive oil, oregano, salt, and pepper and toss to coat well. Transfer to a 9-by-13-inch glass baking dish, reserving the oiled bowl. Roast the cauliflower for 15 to 20 minutes, or until just starting to turn golden brown.

3. Meanwhile, in the same large bowl, combine the olives, spinach, parsley, half the feta, the goat cheese, and the remaining ¼ cup of olive oil. Stir to combine well and incorporate the goat cheese into the mixture.

4. Transfer the hot cauliflower to the large bowl with the olive-and-cheese mixture and toss to coat well. Add the heavy cream and toss again. Transfer back to the baking dish and sprinkle the remaining 4 ounces of feta on top of the vegetables. Return to the oven and roast until bubbly, 10 to 12 minutes. Serve warm.

MACRONUTRIENTS: 82% Fat, 11% Protein, 7% Carbs

PER SERVING: Calories: 414; Total Fat: 38g; Saturated Fat: 16g; Protein: 12g; Total Carbs: 8g; Fiber: 3g; Net Carbs: 5g

Brussels Sprouts with Pancetta and Walnuts

SERVES 4

Prep Time: 10 minutes / **Cook Time:** 40 minutes

Reduces Inflammation

High in anti-inflammatory omega-3 fats, this rich side dish doesn't compromise health for flavor! Roasting is an easy hands-off cooking method that produces a crispy texture—it makes Brussels sprouts irresistible, even if you weren't previously a fan. Feel free to prepare this recipe on the stove top if you prefer. Just panfry the veggies and meat in olive oil over high heat until crispy, then toss with the nuts to finish. This side is also wonderful served with crumbled goat cheese for a really rich dish.

½ cup walnuts

1 pound Brussels sprouts, trimmed and halved

6 tablespoons extra-virgin olive oil, divided

½ teaspoon salt

½ teaspoon garlic powder

¼ teaspoon freshly ground black pepper

4 ounces pancetta, cut into ½-inch strips

2 tablespoons balsamic vinegar

1. Preheat the oven to 425°F. Place the walnuts on a large baking sheet lined with aluminum foil.

2. Toast the walnuts until just browned and fragrant, but not burned, 3 to 4 minutes. Remove from the oven, roughly chop, and set aside, reserving the foil on the baking sheet.

3. In a large bowl, combine the Brussels sprouts, 4 tablespoons of olive oil, the salt, garlic powder, and pepper and toss to coat well.

4. Transfer the Brussels sprouts to the prepared baking sheet. Do not rinse the bowl. Roast the sprouts for 20 minutes. Remove from the oven, sprinkle with the pancetta, and toss to blend. Return to the oven and roast until the sprouts are golden brown and pancetta is crispy, another 10 to 15 minutes. Remove from the oven and return to the reserved bowl.

5. Add the chopped toasted walnuts to the warm Brussels sprouts and pancetta, and toss to coat.

6. In a small bowl, whisk together the remaining 2 tablespoons of olive oil and the vinegar and drizzle over the mixture. Toss to coat and serve warm.

INGREDIENT TIP: Pancetta is an Italian version of bacon. Both are made from cured pork belly, but pancetta is not smoked, giving it a more pure flavor. It is definitely a treat, but if you can't find it at your local grocery, feel free to substitute traditional bacon.

MACRONUTRIENTS: 82% Fat, 8% Protein, 10% Carbs

PER SERVING: Calories: 450; Total Fat: 41g; Saturated Fat: 8g; Protein: 10g; Total Carbs: 14g; Fiber: 5g; Net Carbs: 9g

Garlicky Creamed Spinach

SERVES 4

Prep Time: 5 minutes / **Cook Time:** 15 minutes

Bone Health

Spinach is a great nondairy source of calcium, the mineral essential to bone health, especially as we age. This dish provides a satiating and tasty way to get a good dose of the green leafy vegetable and add some variety into your meals. Serve with a simple grilled steak or salmon fillet for a complete meal.

4 tablespoons
  unsalted butter

½ small onion, minced

4 cloves garlic, minced

1 (16-ounce) package frozen
  spinach (about 4 cups),
  thawed and drained of
  excess water

4 ounces cream cheese,
  room temperature

½ cup heavy cream

1 teaspoon salt

¼ teaspoon freshly ground
  black pepper

¼ teaspoon nutmeg
  (optional)

1. Heat the butter in a medium skillet over low heat. Add the onion and sauté for 3 to 4 minutes, or until starting to turn golden. Add the garlic and sauté for another 1 to 2 minutes, or until fragrant.

2. Add the spinach and sauté for 1 to 2 minutes, or until the water has released.

3. Stir in the softened cream cheese and cook over low heat until melted and well incorporated with the spinach, 2 to 3 minutes.

4. Whisk in the heavy cream, salt, pepper, and nutmeg (if using). Increase heat to medium and cook, whisking constantly, until smooth and creamy, 3 to 4 minutes. Serve warm.

MACRONUTRIENTS: 85% Fat, 6% Protein, 9% Carbs

PER SERVING: Calories: 342; Total Fat: 33g; Saturated Fat: 20g; Protein: 7g; Total Carbs: 9g; Fiber: 4g; Net Carbs: 5g

Roasted Delicata Squash and Kale Salad

SERVES 8

Prep Time: 5 minutes / **Cook Time:** 20 minutes

Reduces Inflammation

The skin on delicata squash is so tender you can eat it—no need to peel. Not only is this a time-saver, but the skin adds extra fiber and nutrients to the dish. Although winter squash are lower in carbohydrates than potatoes or other starchy vegetables, we still have to keep portions small to keep macronutrient ratios in check. In this dish, a little goes a long way, and the added crunch from anti-inflammatory pumpkin seeds makes for a real treat!

1 cup slivered delicata squash half-moons, about ¼ inch thick (see ingredient tip)

6 tablespoons extra-virgin olive oil, divided

1 teaspoon salt, divided

4 cups baby kale or baby spinach leaves

¼ cup roasted pumpkin seeds (or pecans or walnuts)

1 tablespoon balsamic vinegar

¼ teaspoon freshly ground black pepper

4 ounces goat cheese, crumbled

1. Preheat the oven to 400°F and line a rimmed baking sheet with aluminum foil.

2. In a medium bowl, toss together the squash, 2 tablespoons of olive oil, and ½ teaspoon of salt. Spread the squash in a single layer on the prepared baking sheet, reserving the bowl, and roast until golden and tender, 15 to 20 minutes.

3. Meanwhile, place the kale in the reserved bowl. Add the pumpkin seeds. Set aside.

4. In a small bowl, whisk together the remaining 4 tablespoons of olive oil, the remaining ½ teaspoon of salt, the vinegar, and pepper and set aside.

5. When the squash has cooked, remove from the oven and add the warm squash to the greens. Drizzle with the dressing and toss to coat well. Top with goat cheese and serve warm.

PREP TIP: To prepare the squash, cut the delicata in half lengthwise and remove the seeds. Cut into half-moons about ¼ inch thick, keeping the skin intact.

MACRONUTRIENTS: 82% Fat, 10% Protein, 8% Carbs

PER SERVING: Calories: 162; Total Fat: 15g; Saturated Fat: 4g; Protein: 4g; Total Carbs: 4g; Fiber: 1g; Net Carbs: 3g

Sausage Balls

MAKES 2 dozen (2 balls per serving)
Prep Time: 5 minutes / **Cook Time:** 25 minutes

These savory sausage balls are great as an appetizer for a party or even just a quick and easy snack. This recipe makes a large batch for entertaining, but extra sausage balls will freeze well in a freezer-safe bag for up to 3 months.

1 pound bulk Italian sausage (not sweet)

1 cup almond flour

1½ cups finely shredded cheddar cheese

1 large egg

2 teaspoons baking powder

1 teaspoon onion powder

1 teaspoon fennel seed (optional)

½ teaspoon cayenne pepper (optional)

1. Preheat the oven to 350°F and line a rimmed baking sheet with aluminum foil.

2. In a large bowl, combine all the ingredients. Use a fork to mix until well blended.

3. Form the sausage mixture into 1½-inch balls and place 1 inch apart on the prepared baking sheet.

4. Bake for 20 to 25 minutes, or until browned and cooked through.

MACRONUTRIENTS: 77% Fat, 19% Protein, 4% Carbs

PER SERVING: Calories: 241; Total Fat: 21g; Saturated Fat: 7g; Protein: 11g; Total Carbs: 3g; Fiber: 1g; Net Carbs: 2g

Bacon-Studded Pimento Cheese

SERVES 6
Prep Time: 10 minutes, plus 30 minutes to chill
Cook Time: 5 minutes

Bone Health

Filled with calcium, this savory cheese dish is a flavorful and keto-friendly way to snack. On its own, cheese has higher ratios of protein and needs to be paired with a pure fat to keep ketogenic ratios in check. Adding the mayonnaise and cream cheese does just this and makes this Southern dish the perfect keto-friendly treat!

2 ounces bacon (about
    4 thick slices)
4 ounces cream cheese,
    room temperature
¼ cup mayonnaise
¼ teaspoon onion powder
¼ teaspoon cayenne pepper
    (optional)
1 cup thick-shredded
    extra-sharp
    cheddar cheese
2 ounces jarred diced
    pimentos, drained

1. Chop the raw bacon into ½-inch-thick pieces. Cook in a small skillet over medium heat until crispy, 3 to 4 minutes. Use a slotted spoon to transfer the bacon onto a layer of paper towels. Reserve the rendered fat.

2. In a large bowl, combine the cream cheese, mayonnaise, onion powder, and cayenne (if using), and beat with an electric mixer or by hand until smooth and creamy.

3. Add the rendered bacon fat, cheddar cheese, and pimentos and mix until well combined.

4. Refrigerate for at least 30 minutes before serving to allow flavors to blend. Serve cold with raw veggies such as celery, cucumber, or radish—or mixed into Pimento Cheese Scrambled Eggs (page 56).

INGREDIENT TIP: You can buy thick-shredded cheese in many grocery stores, but you can achieve the same texture by shredding a block of cheese using a box grater. A finer shred will taste fine, but won't have the same texture.

MACRONUTRIENTS: 82% Fat, 14% Protein, 4% Carbs

PER SERVING: Calories: 216; Total Fat: 20g; Saturated Fat: 8g; Protein: 8g; Total Carbs: 2g; Fiber: 0g; Net Carbs: 2g

Spinach and Artichoke Dip

SERVES 8

Prep Time: 5 minutes / **Cook Time:** 25 minutes

Freezer-Friendly

This is my go-to appetizer when entertaining. I serve it with raw veggies such as celery, bell peppers, cucumber, and endive spears. Leftover dip is delicious mixed into scrambled eggs the next morning or served over a leaner grilled chicken or fish, which boosts the fats.

4 tablespoons extra-virgin olive oil, divided

½ small yellow onion, diced

1 cup drained artichoke hearts, chopped (about half of a 14-ounce can)

8 ounces frozen spinach, thawed and drained of excess liquid (about 2 cups)

1 teaspoon salt

½ to 1 teaspoon red pepper flakes

½ teaspoon garlic powder

8 ounces cream cheese, room temperature

½ cup shredded Parmesan cheese, divided

½ cup mayonnaise

1. Preheat the oven to 375°F. Drizzle 2 tablespoons of olive oil in an 8-inch square glass baking dish and swirl to coat the bottom and sides.

2. Heat the remaining 2 tablespoons of olive oil in a medium skillet over medium heat. Add the onion and artichoke hearts and sauté for 3 to 4 minutes, or until the onion is soft and lightly browned. Add the spinach, salt, red pepper flakes, and garlic powder and sauté for another 1 to 2 minutes.

3. Add the softened cream cheese and cook, stirring constantly, until cheese is fully melted and well incorporated into the vegetables. Add ¼ cup of Parmesan cheese and stir until melted, another 1 to 2 minutes.

4. Remove the skillet from heat and mix in the mayonnaise. Transfer the mixture to the prepared baking dish, and sprinkle the top with the remaining ¼ cup of Parmesan cheese. Bake uncovered until bubbly and the cheese on the top has melted, 10 to 12 minutes. Serve warm.

VARIATION TIP: To really jazz this up, you can add lump crabmeat or chopped cooked shrimp in with the mayonnaise before baking for a presentation-worthy appetizer.

MACRONUTRIENTS: 86% Fat, 7% Protein, 7% Carbs

PER SERVING: Calories: 298; Total Fat: 29g; Saturated Fat: 9g; Protein: 6g; Total Carbs: 6g; Fiber: 3g; Net Carbs: 3g

Crunchy Granola Bars

MAKES 16 bars (1 bar per serving)
Prep Time: 15 minutes / **Cook Time:** 15 minutes

Freezer-Friendly

Most store-bought granola bars are loaded with sugars, hidden carbs, and inflammatory fats—in short, they're more like a candy bar than a healthy snack. These bars are a keto-friendly and tasty homemade option with nice crunch. This recipe makes a big batch, so store some in the freezer for a great on-the-go snack or grab two for a quick breakfast. They are also wonderful crumbled over plain yogurt. Feel free to mix up the flavor using any nut, seed, or nut butter (such as macadamia or cashew) you may have on hand.

½ cup unsweetened almond butter

2 tablespoons coconut oil

2 to 4 tablespoons granulated sugar-free sweetener

1 egg white

1 teaspoon ground cinnamon

1 teaspoon vanilla extract

¼ teaspoon salt

2 tablespoons almond flour

1 cup unsweetened coconut flakes

1 cup slivered almonds

1 cup chopped roasted unsalted pecans

1 cup shelled pumpkin seeds

1. Preheat the oven to 350°F. Line an 8-inch square glass baking dish with parchment paper, letting the paper hang over the sides.

2. In a large glass bowl, combine the almond butter, coconut oil, and sweetener and microwave for 30 seconds, or until the coconut oil is melted.

3. Whisk in the egg white, cinnamon, vanilla extract, and salt until smooth and creamy.

4. Stir in the almond flour, coconut flakes, almonds, pecans, and pumpkin seeds until thoroughly combined.

5. Transfer the mixture into the prepared dish and press down firmly with a spatula to cover the bottom evenly.

6. Bake for 15 minutes, or until crispy and slightly browned around the edges.

7. Allow to cool completely before cutting into 16 bars. Bars can be stored tightly wrapped in the freezer for up to 3 months.

MACRONUTRIENTS: 78% Fat, 11% Protein, 11% Carbs

PER SERVING: Calories: 215; Total Fat: 20g; Saturated Fat: 5g; Protein: 6g; Total Carbs: 6g; Fiber: 3g; Net Carbs: 3g

Pecan Sandy Fat Bombs

MAKES 8 (1 fat bomb per serving)
Prep Time: 15 minutes, plus 1 hour to chill

Brain Health

Fat bombs are a delicious and convenient way to get extra fat in a leaner meal or as a satiating snack. These help promote ketone production, which increases energy and mental clarity. Added bonus: They taste just like pecan sandy cookie dough. What's not to love?

½ cup (1 stick) unsalted butter, room temperature

¼ cup granulated sugar-free sweetener

½ teaspoon vanilla extract

1 cup almond flour

¾ cup chopped roasted unsalted pecans, divided

1. In a large bowl, use an electric mixer on medium speed to cream together the butter and sweetener until smooth. Add the vanilla and beat well.

2. Add the almond flour and ½ cup of chopped pecans, and stir until well incorporated. Place the mixture in the refrigerator for 30 minutes, or until slightly hardened. Meanwhile, very finely chop the remaining ¼ cup of pecans.

3. Using a spoon or your hands, form the chilled mixture into 8 (1-inch) round balls and place on a baking sheet lined with parchment paper. Roll each ball in the finely chopped pecans, and refrigerate for at least 30 minutes before serving. Store in an airtight container in the refrigerator for up to 1 week or in the freezer for up to 2 months.

MACRONUTRIENTS: 88% Fat, 5% Protein, 7% Carbs

PER SERVING: Calories: 242; Total Fat: 25g; Saturated Fat: 8g; Protein: 4g; Total Carbs: 4g; Fiber: 3g; Net Carbs: 1g

Almond and Chocolate Chia Pudding

SERVES 4

Prep Time: 10 minutes, plus 6 hours to chill

Reduces Inflammation

Reminiscent of tapioca pudding, this chia pudding makes for a great snack or light breakfast. Chia seeds are high in anti-inflammatory omega-3 fatty acids, as well as fiber for digestive health. This dish will store in the refrigerator for up to a week, so make a batch at the beginning of the week and enjoy whenever you need a tasty treat.

1 (14-ounce) can full-fat coconut milk

⅓ cup chia seeds

1 tablespoon unsweetened cocoa powder

2 tablespoons unsweetened almond butter

2 to 3 teaspoons granulated sugar-free sweetener of choice (optional)

½ teaspoon vanilla extract

½ teaspoon almond extract (optional)

1. Combine all the ingredients in a small bowl, whisking well to fully incorporate the almond butter.

2. Divide the mixture between four ramekins or small glass jars.

3. Cover and refrigerate for at least 6 hours, preferably overnight. Serve cold.

INGREDIENT TIP: For the best texture and macro profile, make sure you use canned full-fat coconut milk, not refrigerated lighter coconut or coconut-almond blend.

MACRONUTRIENTS: 78% Fat, 7% Protein, 15% Carbs

PER SERVING: Calories: 335; Total Fat: 31g; Saturated Fat: 20g; Protein: 7g; Total Carbs: 13g; Fiber: 7g; Net Carbs: 6g

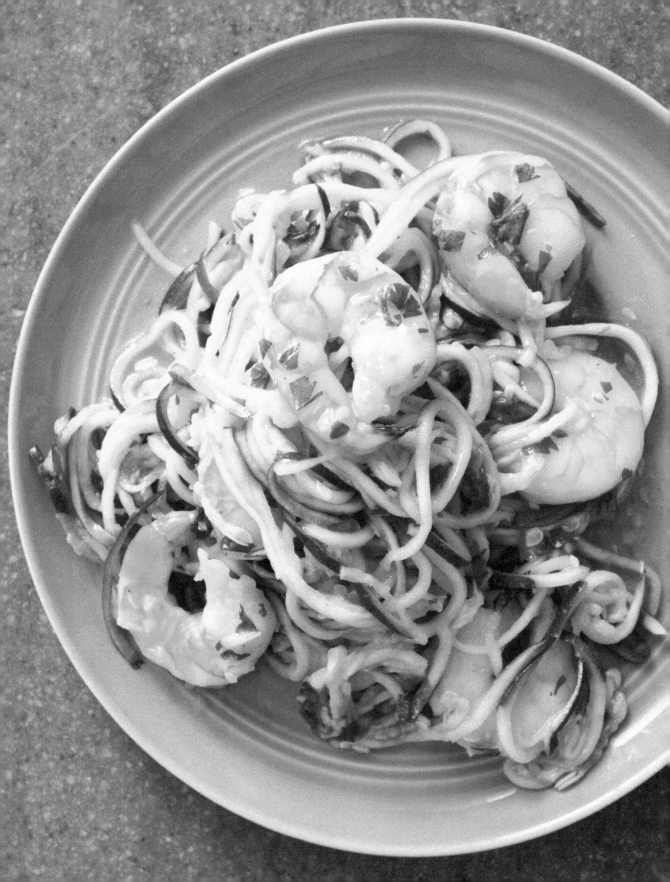

CHAPTER SIX

Seafood & Poultry

Shrimp and Chicken Gumbo

SERVES 6

Prep Time: 15 minutes / **Cook Time:** 40 minutes

Gumbo and jambalaya are close cousins, with roots in Cajun and Creole cuisine. Traditional jambalaya has rice cooked in with the meat, seafood, and vegetables, whereas gumbo is served over the rice. This keto-friendly gumbo recipe, full of veggies and protein, is hearty enough to stand on its own and needs no accompaniment!

For the gumbo

- ½ cup extra-virgin olive oil, divided
- ½ pound andouille sausage links, sliced ¼ inch thick
- ½ small yellow onion, chopped
- 1 red bell pepper, stemmed and seeded, finely chopped
- 2 ribs celery, cut into ¼-inch-thick half-moons
- 8 ounces boneless, skinless chicken thighs (about 2 thighs), cut into ½-inch cubes
- 1 (14½-ounce) can diced tomatoes, with juice
- 1 cup chicken stock
- 1 teaspoon salt
- 1 tablespoon Creole seasoning blend (see ingredient tip)
- 8 ounces peeled and deveined shrimp

1. **To make the gumbo.** Heat 2 tablespoons of olive oil in a large skillet over medium-high heat. Add the sausage and cook until browned on all sides, 3 to 4 minutes. Using a slotted spoon, remove the sausage from the pan and cover to keep warm.

2. Add an additional 2 tablespoons of olive oil to the skillet and reduce heat to medium. Add the onion, bell pepper, and celery to the skillet and sauté until the vegetables are just tender, 4 to 5 minutes, stirring frequently.

3. Add the chicken and sauté until browned, 2 to 3 minutes. Add in the tomatoes and their juice, stock, remaining ¼ cup of olive oil, salt, and Creole seasoning. Reduce the heat to low, and cook, covered, for 15 to 18 minutes, or until fragrant and the chicken is cooked through.

4. Remove the skillet from the heat, add the cooked sausage and raw shrimp, and stir to incorporate. Cover and let sit 5 minutes to cook the shrimp in the hot liquid.

For the avocado mayo

1 large ripe avocado, pitted and peeled

¼ cup mayonnaise

Juice of 1 lemon

½ teaspoon salt

⅛ teaspoon cayenne pepper (optional)

5. **To make the avocado mayo.** In a medium bowl, mash the avocado well with a fork. Whisk in the mayonnaise, lemon juice, salt, and cayenne pepper (if using) until smooth.

6. Divide the gumbo into six bowls and top each with 2 tablespoons of avocado mayo.

INGREDIENT TIP: Creole seasoning can be found in the spice aisle of most grocery stores, but you can make your own by blending together 1 tablespoon of smoked paprika, ½ teaspoon of garlic powder, ½ teaspoon of onion powder, ½ teaspoon of dried thyme, ½ teaspoon of dried oregano, and ¼ teaspoon of cayenne pepper.

MACRONUTRIENTS: 75% Fat, 20% Protein, 5% Carbs

PER SERVING: Calories: 485; Total Fat: 41g; Saturated Fat: 8g; Protein: 23g; Total Carbs: 8g; Fiber: 4g; Net Carbs: 4g

Clam Chowder

SERVES 4

Prep Time: 5 minutes / **Cook Time:** 15 minutes

Freezer-Friendly

Warm, creamy chowders are the ultimate in comfort food. Higher-fat traditional clam chowder misses the keto mark with the inclusion of potatoes or other starchy vegetables and flour in the base. This version uses chopped cauliflower in place of the potato, and cream cheese to thicken the base—it really works! For a real treat, serve with a Keto Biscuit (see the Biscuit-Topped Chicken Pot Pie recipe, page 92).

4 slices bacon, chopped into ½-inch squares

2 tablespoons unsalted butter

½ small yellow onion, chopped

4 ribs celery, cut into ¼-inch-thick half-moons

1 cup chopped cauliflower florets, cut to about ½ inch thick

4 ounces chopped mushrooms

4 cloves garlic, minced

1 teaspoon dried tarragon

1 teaspoon salt

¼ teaspoon freshly ground black pepper

8 ounces bottled clam juice

1 cup vegetable stock or broth

½ cup heavy cream

8 ounces cream cheese, room temperature

3 (6½-ounce) cans chopped clams, with juice

¼ cup freshly chopped Italian parsley

1. Place the bacon in a medium saucepan over medium heat. Fry until just browned and most of the fat has been rendered, 3 to 4 minutes. Remove the bacon with a slotted spoon, reserving the rendered fat.

2. Add the butter to the pan with the fat and melt over medium heat. Add the onion, celery, cauliflower, and mushrooms and sauté until vegetables are just tender, 4 to 5 minutes. Add the garlic, tarragon, salt, and pepper and sauté for another 30 seconds or until fragrant.

3. Add the clam juice, stock, cream, and cream cheese and whisk until the cheese is melted and creamy, 2 to 3 minutes. Add the clams and their juice, bring to a simmer, and cook for 1 to 2 minutes so the flavors meld. Stir in the parsley and serve warm.

MACRONUTRIENTS: 72% Fat, 20% Protein, 8% Carbs

PER SERVING: Calories: 671; Total Fat: 54g; Saturated Fat: 29g; Protein: 34g; Total Carbs: 15g; Fiber: 2g; Net Carbs: 13g

Shrimp Scampi with Zucchini Noodles

SERVES 4

Prep Time: 5 minutes / **Cook Time:** 10 minutes

Protein Power

Traditional scampi contains mostly butter, and while butter is healthy in moderation, it is all saturated fat. This version uses more olive oil than butter, making it heart-healthy, anti-inflammatory, and loaded with protein. The warm sauce will "cook" the zucchini without making it soggy, so be sure your zoodles are fresh.

½ cup extra-virgin olive oil, divided

1 pound shrimp, peeled and deveined

1 teaspoon salt

¼ teaspoon freshly ground black pepper

2 tablespoons unsalted butter

6 garlic cloves, minced

2 tablespoons dry white wine or chicken broth

½ teaspoon red pepper flakes

Zest and juice of 1 lemon

¼ cup chopped fresh Italian parsley

4 cups spiralized zucchini noodles (about 2 medium zucchini)

1. In a large skillet, heat ¼ cup of olive oil over medium-high heat. Add the shrimp, sprinkle with salt and pepper, and sauté for 2 to 3 minutes, or until the shrimp is just pink. Using a slotted spoon, transfer the shrimp to a bowl and cover to keep warm.

2. Reduce heat to low and add the remaining ¼ cup of olive oil, butter, and garlic. Cook the garlic, stirring frequently, until very fragrant, 3 to 4 minutes.

3. Whisk in the wine, red pepper flakes, and lemon zest and juice. Increase the heat to medium-high and bring to a simmer. Remove the skillet from the heat as soon as the liquid simmers. Return the shrimp to the skillet, add the parsley, and toss.

4. To serve, place the raw zucchini noodles in a large bowl. Add the shrimp and sauce and toss to coat.

VARIATION TIP: For an extra boost of veggies, add a few handfuls of spinach to the raw zucchini noodles before tossing with the sauce and shrimp.

MACRONUTRIENTS: 72% Fat, 23% Protein, 5% Carbs

PER SERVING: Calories: 414; Total Fat: 34g; Saturated Fat: 8g; Protein: 25g; Total Carbs: 5g; Fiber: 2g; Net Carbs: 3g

Parchment-Baked Cod and Asparagus with Beurre Blanc

SERVES 4

Prep Time: 15 minutes / **Cook Time:** 15 minutes

Protein Power

Beurre blanc is a classic French sauce made by emulsifying butter with vinegar or white wine. Julia Child popularized this sauce in America. It goes well with almost any fish or vegetable, but my favorite way to serve it is with a buttery white flaky fish such as cod or halibut, and some delicate asparagus. Baking the fish and vegetables together in parchment keeps the fish tender and minimizes cleanup—win-win! Slather both with the rich sauce and you'll have an easy dinner that feels just like a French restaurant specialty.

1 pound skinless cod, halibut, or other white flaky fish

1 teaspoon salt, divided

½ teaspoon freshly ground black pepper, divided

2 garlic cloves, thinly sliced

1 lemon, thinly sliced

½ pound asparagus spears, rough ends trimmed

4 tablespoons extra-virgin olive oil, divided

1 tablespoon finely chopped red onion

¼ cup white wine vinegar

¼ cup heavy cream

½ cup (1 stick) chilled unsalted butter, cut into tablespoon-size pieces

1. Preheat the oven to 375°F.

2. Place 1 large sheet of parchment paper (about twice the size of the fish fillet) on a rimmed baking sheet. Place the fish in the center of the parchment and sprinkle with ½ teaspoon of the salt and ¼ teaspoon of the pepper.

3. Top the fish with the garlic and lemon slices. Top with the asparagus spears and drizzle with 2 tablespoons of olive oil.

4. Top the fish with a second large piece of parchment. Starting on a long side, fold the paper up to about 1 inch from the fish and vegetables. Repeat on the remaining sides, going in a clockwise direction. Fold in each corner once to secure.

5. Bake for 10 to 12 minutes, until the fish is cooked through and flakes easily when poked with a paring knife.

6. Meanwhile, prepare the sauce. Heat the remaining 2 tablespoons of olive oil over medium heat. Add the red onion and sauté until tender, 3 to 4 minutes. Add the vinegar, cream, remaining ½ teaspoon of salt, and ¼ teaspoon of pepper. Bring to a simmer and reduce heat to low.

7. Whisking constantly, add the butter, a couple tablespoons at a time, until melted and creamy. Remove the sauce from the heat and serve warm, poured over the fish and asparagus.

MACRONUTRIENTS: 80% Fat, 17% Protein, 3% Carbs

PER SERVING: Calories: 472; Total Fat: 43g; Saturated Fat: 19g; Protein: 19g; Total Carbs: 4g; Fiber: 1g; Net Carbs: 3g

Coconut-Crusted Salmon with Avocado Sauce

SERVES 4

Prep Time: 20 minutes / **Cook Time:** 20 minutes

Reduces Inflammation

So many of my patients tell me they'd love to eat more salmon, but just can't master cooking it. This recipe is incredibly forgiving and will convert even a non–salmon lover. Full of anti-inflammatory omega-3 fatty acids from the salmon, avocado, and flaxseed, this recipe scores a home run on nutrition. You can also serve this with Versatile Tartar Sauce (page 127).

¼ cup melted coconut oil, divided

⅓ cup coconut flour

1½ teaspoons salt, divided

1 large egg

½ cup unsweetened flaked coconut

¼ cup ground flaxseed

4 (4-ounce) skinless salmon fillets

1 very ripe avocado, pitted and peeled

1 tablespoon fresh lime juice (from about ½ of a lime)

¼ cup full-fat canned coconut milk, plus more as needed

1. Preheat the oven to 375°F. Line a baking sheet with aluminum foil and coat with 2 tablespoons of coconut oil.

2. Set out three shallow bowls. Combine the coconut flour and 1 teaspoon of salt in the first, whisk the egg in the second, and combine the flaked coconut and flaxseed in the third.

3. To coat the fish, dredge each salmon fillet first in the coconut flour mixture, then the egg, and last the flaked coconut mixture. Place onto the prepared baking sheet and drizzle the fillets with the remaining 2 tablespoons of the melted coconut oil. Bake for 15 to 18 minutes, or until the fish is tender and the coconut crust is golden brown.

4. While the salmon bakes, prepare the sauce. In a food processor or blender, combine the avocado, lime juice, remaining ½ teaspoon of salt, and the coconut milk. (You can also use an immersion blender.) Blend until smooth, adding more coconut milk if the mixture is very thick. It should be the consistency of sour cream.

5. Serve the salmon warm with the avocado sauce.

MACRONUTRIENTS: 70% Fat, 22% Protein, 8% Carbs

PER SERVING: Calories: 550; Total Fat: 45g; Saturated Fat: 23g; Protein: 29g; Total Carbs: 11g; Fiber: 7g; Net Carbs: 4g

Baked Buffalo Chicken Wings

SERVES 8

Prep Time: 10 minutes / **Cook Time:** 50 minutes

Protein Power

Wings aren't just for sports bars! Once you realize how easy these are to make at home, they'll be on your weekly rotation, like they are at my house. You can adapt the sauce to make it less spicy for milder wings, or use different spices in the rub and sauce, such as curry, chili powder, ginger, or oregano.

1 tablespoon extra-virgin olive oil

1 tablespoon smoked paprika

1 tablespoon chili powder

2 teaspoons onion powder

2 teaspoons garlic powder, divided

1 teaspoon salt

4 pounds chicken wings

½ cup (1 stick) unsalted butter

½ cup hot sauce (such as Tabasco or Frank's RedHot)

2 teaspoons white vinegar

1 teaspoon Worcestershire sauce

½ cup blue cheese or ranch dressing (no sugar added) for serving

1. Preheat the oven to 450°F. Line a large rimmed baking sheet with aluminum foil. Place a wire rack or slotted broiler pan over the foil and rub the rack with the olive oil.

2. In a large bowl, combine the paprika, chili powder, onion powder, 1 teaspoon of garlic powder, and salt, and stir well. Add the chicken wings and toss to coat. Place the wings in a single layer on the prepared wire rack and bake until the skin is golden brown and crispy, 40 to 45 minutes. Wash and rinse the bowl and reserve for later use.

3. Meanwhile, prepare the sauce. Melt the butter in a small saucepan over low heat. Whisk in the hot sauce, vinegar, Worcestershire sauce, and remaining 1 teaspoon of garlic powder until smooth. Transfer to the reserved bowl and cover to keep warm.

4. When the wings have finished cooking, remove them from the oven and toss with the buffalo sauce in the bowl until well coated. Return to the wire rack and bake at 450°F for an additional 5 minutes.

5. Serve the wings warm with dressing for dipping.

MACRONUTRIENTS: 75% Fat, 22% Protein, 3% Carbs

PER SERVING: Calories: 408; Total Fat: 34g; Saturated Fat: 10g; Protein: 22g; Total Carbs: 3g; Fiber: 1g; Net Carbs: 2g

Stir-Fried Chicken and Broccoli with Cashews

SERVES 4

Prep Time: 10 minutes / **Cook Time:** 20 minutes

Reduces Inflammation

Most bottled stir-fry sauces are loaded with sugars, and many contain inflammatory fats. The sauce in this recipe uses homemade Cashew Hummus (page 122) or almond butter, filling it with flavor and inflammation-reducing, heart-healthy fats from nuts, seeds, and olive oil. Garlic and ginger also have wonderful anti-inflammatory properties, making this dish a home run health-wise and flavor-wise.

¼ cup Cashew Hummus (page 122) or unsweetened almond butter

2 tablespoons soy sauce

1 tablespoon sesame oil

1 tablespoon rice wine vinegar

1 teaspoon ground ginger

4 tablespoons extra-virgin olive oil, divided

1 pound boneless, skinless chicken thighs, cut into ½-inch cubes

4 cloves garlic, minced

½ small yellow onion, diced

1 tablespoon chopped fresh ginger

2 cups broccoli crowns, cut into 1-inch florets

¼ cup whole unsalted cashews (raw or roasted)

Cauliflower Fried Rice (page 121), for serving

¼ cup sesame seeds

1. In a small bowl, whisk the cashew hummus, soy sauce, sesame oil, vinegar, and ground ginger and set aside.

2. Heat 2 tablespoons of olive oil in a large skillet over medium-high heat. Add the chicken and sauté until browned, 4 to 5 minutes. Add the garlic and sauté for another 30 seconds. Transfer the browned chicken to a bowl and cover to keep warm.

3. Heat the remaining 2 tablespoons of olive oil in the same skillet over medium heat. Add the onion and fresh ginger and sauté for 2 minutes. Add the broccoli and sauté, stirring frequently, until just tender and lightly browned, 4 to 5 minutes.

4. Return the browned chicken to the skillet and pour in the reserved cashew sauce, stirring to coat the vegetables and chicken. Reduce heat to low, cover, and cook until the vegetables are very tender and chicken is cooked through, another 4 to 5 minutes. Remove from heat and stir in the whole cashews.

5. Serve over Cauliflower Fried Rice, sprinkled with the sesame seeds.

MACRONUTRIENTS: 68% Fat, 23% Protein, 9% Carbs

PER SERVING: Calories: 607; Total Fat: 47g; Saturated Fat: 7g; Protein: 34g; Total Carbs: 16g; Fiber: 6g; Net Carbs: 10g

Cheesy Chicken and Broccoli Casserole

SERVES 6

Prep Time: 10 minutes, plus 5 minutes to rest
Cook Time: 30 minutes

Freezer-Friendly

Creamy and cheesy, this hearty casserole is sure to please everyone. It freezes wonderfully, so I suggest doubling the recipe to keep one for a busy week down the line. I love chicken thighs for their moisture and fat content, but you can substitute breasts or canned chicken here if you prefer, as the fat from the other ingredients will offset the leaner protein.

¼ cup extra-virgin olive oil

1 pound chicken thighs, cut into small cubes, about ½ inch thick

2 cups broccoli florets, cut into small pieces, about ½ inch thick

1 teaspoon salt, divided

½ teaspoon freshly ground black pepper, divided

¼ cup chicken stock

¼ cup heavy cream

8 ounces cream cheese, room temperature

2 cups shredded cheddar cheese, divided

½ cup sour cream

2 teaspoons garlic powder

2 teaspoons onion powder

¼ cup slivered almonds

1. Preheat the oven to 375°F.

2. Heat the olive oil in a large skillet over medium-high heat. Add the chicken, broccoli, ½ teaspoon of salt, and ¼ teaspoon of pepper and sauté until just tender and chicken is browned on all sides, 4 to 5 minutes. Transfer the mixture to an 8-inch square glass baking dish.

3. Combine the stock, cream, and cream cheese in a microwave-safe bowl and microwave on high for 60 to 90 seconds, or until the cream cheese is melted. Add 1 cup of cheddar cheese and stir to combine well.

4. Stir the sour cream, garlic powder, onion powder, remaining ½ teaspoon of salt, and ¼ teaspoon of pepper into the cheese mixture and pour over the broccoli and chicken. Top with the remaining 1 cup of cheddar cheese and the slivered almonds and bake for 20 to 25 minutes, or until bubbly and golden brown. Let rest for 5 minutes before serving.

MACRONUTRIENTS: 79% Fat, 17% Protein, 4% Carbs

PER SERVING: Calories: 643; Total Fat: 57g; Saturated Fat: 24g; Protein: 26g; Total Carbs: 7g; Fiber: 2g; Net Carbs: 5g

Biscuit-Topped Chicken Pot Pie

SERVES 4

Prep Time: 25 minutes / **Cook Time:** 30 minutes

Freezer-Friendly

The cobblestone biscuit topping in this tasty pot pie allows for portioning of the biscuits to keep ratios keto-friendly. This dish can be fully cooked and frozen for an easy go-to midweek dinner on a busy day. Just prepare the pie as directed, cool completely, and cover before freezing for up to 3 months.

For the biscuits

1 cup almond flour

1½ teaspoons baking powder

½ teaspoon salt

2 tablespoons cold butter, diced into small chunks

2 tablespoons heavy cream

1 large egg

2 ounces shredded mozzarella or cheddar cheese

1. Preheat the oven to 375°F.

2. **To make the biscuits.** In a large bowl, combine the almond flour, baking powder, and salt in a large bowl and mix well. Add the cubed butter and use a fork or your hands to crumble it into the flour mixture until it resembles coarse pebbles.

3. Whisk in the heavy cream, 1 tablespoon at a time. Whisk in the egg and cheese until the mixture forms a smooth dough. Set aside.

4. **To make the filling.** Heat the olive oil in a large skillet over medium-high heat. Add the onion, celery, mushrooms, carrot, thyme, salt, and pepper and sauté until vegetables are just tender, 5 to 6 minutes. Add the garlic and sauté for an additional 30 seconds.

5. Add the wine or stock, stirring until most of the liquid has evaporated. Whisk in ¾ cup of heavy cream, and bring to just below a simmer. Reduce heat to low and cook, stirring occasionally, for 4 to 5 minutes.

6. In a microwave-safe bowl, combine the remaining ¼ cup of heavy cream, cream cheese, and Worcestershire sauce and microwave on high for 45 to 60 seconds, or until the cream cheese is melted. Whisk until smooth. Add the cream mixture to the vegetable mixture, stirring until smooth.

For the filling

2 tablespoons extra-virgin olive oil

½ small yellow onion, finely chopped

4 ribs celery, diced small (about 1 cup diced celery)

4 ounces chopped mushrooms

¼ cup diced carrot (about 1 small carrot)

1½ teaspoons dried thyme

1 teaspoon salt

¼ teaspoon freshly ground black pepper

4 cloves garlic, minced

¼ cup dry white wine or chicken stock

1 cup heavy cream, divided

4 ounces cream cheese, room temperature

1 teaspoon Worcestershire sauce

2 cups (4 or 5 thighs) cooked chicken thigh meat, diced

7. Add the diced chicken and stir to combine. Pour the chicken-and-vegetable mixture into an 8-inch square glass baking dish or pie pan.

8. Form the biscuit dough into 8 balls (the mixture will be sticky), flatten into 8 flat biscuits, and place atop the chicken and vegetables. Bake until bubbly and biscuits are golden brown, 16 to 18 minutes.

MAKE-AHEAD TIP: The biscuit dough can be prepared ahead of time and frozen, as well as used in other recipes such as Biscuits and Gravy (page 58) or to accompany soups or stews.

MACRONUTRIENTS: 77% Fat, 17% Protein, 6% Carbs

PER SERVING: Calories: 776; Total Fat: 68g; Saturated Fat: 29g; Protein: 32g; Total Carbs: 13g; Fiber: 4g; Net Carbs: 9g

Slow Cooker White Chicken Chili

SERVES 8

Prep Time: 10 minutes / **Cook Time:** 4½ hours

Protein Power

Most white chilis rely on beans for bulk, but beans are loaded with carbs, so this recipe adapts all the great chili flavors into a keto-friendly, low-carb alternative. With added protein and skin-health power from the collagen in the bone broth, this dish is filling and satisfying, and packs a nutritional punch. I love using my slow cooker whenever I can to save time, but this can also be prepared on the stove top (see variation tip).

¼ cup extra-virgin olive oil

1 small yellow onion, diced

2 pounds boneless, skinless chicken thighs (about 8)

4 to 6 cloves garlic, finely minced

2 cups chicken bone broth

½ cup heavy cream

2 (4-ounce) cans diced mild green chiles

2 teaspoons cumin

2 teaspoons dried oregano

1½ teaspoons salt

½ teaspoon ground coriander

¼ to ½ teaspoon cayenne pepper

2 (8-ounce) blocks cream cheese, room temperature

2 limes, cut into wedges

½ cup chopped cilantro

2 ripe avocados, pitted, peeled, and sliced

1. Heat the olive oil in a large skillet over medium-high heat. Add the onion and chicken thighs and sauté until browned, about 5 minutes. Add garlic and sauté for 30 seconds more, stirring frequently.

2. Transfer the mixture to the bowl of a slow cooker, and add the bone broth, heavy cream, chiles, cumin, oregano, salt, coriander, and cayenne pepper. Cover and cook on low for 4 hours, or until the chicken is cooked through and shreds easily with a fork.

3. Remove the thighs from the slow cooker and place in a large bowl. Using two forks, shred well, and return to the slow cooker.

4. Ladle out ½ cup of the broth into a large bowl. Add the cream cheese to the broth and stir until smooth. Transfer back to the slow cooker and cook on low, whisking occasionally, until very creamy and any remaining lumps of cream cheese have melted completely, another 15 to 20 minutes.

5. Serve the chili warm garnished with lime wedges, cilantro, and avocado slices.

VARIATION TIP: Cut the chicken into bite-size pieces. Heat the oil in a stock pot over medium-high heat. Add the onion and sauté for 4 to 5 minutes. Add the chicken and brown on all sides. Microwave together cream cheese and ½ cup of stock. Whisk until creamy. Add to the chicken, reduce heat to low, and simmer until chicken is cooked through, 10 to 12 minutes.

MACRONUTRIENTS: 72% Fat, 21% Protein, 7% Carbs

PER SERVING: Calories: 540; Total Fat: 44g; Saturated Fat: 18g; Protein: 28g; Total Carbs: 11g; Fiber: 4g; Net Carbs: 7g

Baked Spaghetti Squash Carbonara with Chicken

SERVES 6

Freezer-Friendly

Prep Time: 15 minutes, plus 10 minutes to cool
Cook Time: 40 minutes

With only 10g carbs per cup, spaghetti squash is a great pasta substitute utilized on many low-carb diets. However, it is still considered a "starchy veggie," so quantities must be limited on a ketogenic diet. Have no fear, though; this recipe achieves a perfect balance of flavor, texture, and nutrition while remaining keto-friendly. Take care not to overcook the squash or it will be mushy. This dish freezes well, so consider doubling the recipe and saving a batch for later.

1 small spaghetti squash

½ cup extra-virgin olive oil, divided

6 ounces thick-cut bacon (preferably nitrate-free), cut into ½-inch-thick strips

1 pound boneless, skinless chicken thighs, cut into ½-inch cubes

4 garlic cloves, minced

3 large egg yolks

½ cup heavy cream

1 cup freshly grated Parmesan cheese, divided

¼ teaspoon freshly ground black pepper

¼ cup fresh Italian parsley, chopped

1. Preheat the oven to 400°F. With a very sharp knife, cut the spaghetti squash in half lengthwise. Scoop out all the seeds (see ingredient tip), and coat the cut sides of the squash with 1 tablespoon of oil per side.

2. Place squash halves cut-side down in a 9-by-13-inch glass baking dish and roast until just barely tender, 20 to 25 minutes. Remove from the oven and flip the halves to cut-side up and allow to cool for 10 minutes.

3. Meanwhile, prepare the filling. Cook the bacon in a large skillet over medium heat and fry until crispy and fat has been rendered, 4 to 5 minutes.

4. Using a slotted spoon, transfer the cooked bacon to a large bowl and cover to keep warm, reserving the rendered fat.

5. Add the remaining 2 tablespoons of olive oil to the fat in the skillet and heat over medium heat. Sauté the cubed chicken until golden and cooked through, stirring frequently, 5 to 6 minutes. Add the minced garlic and sauté for another 30 seconds.

6. Transfer the cooked chicken, garlic, and all the cooking fat to the bowl with the cooked bacon, and cover.

7. In a small bowl, beat together the egg yolks, heavy cream, ¼ cup of Parmesan, and pepper. Set aside.

8. When the cooked squash is just cool enough to handle, but still very warm (you can use potholders to handle the squash), use a fork to gently scrape the cooked flesh in rows to form long pasta-like strings and place in a large bowl. Reserve the baking dish and keep the oven on. Add the remaining ¼ cup of olive oil to the squash and toss to coat well.

9. Tossing with tongs, slowly pour the egg-and-cream mixture onto the warm squash, tossing until the eggs thicken and the cheese melts. Add the cooked bacon, chicken, and reserved fats, and toss to coat well.

10. Transfer the squash mixture and sauce to the glass baking dish, top with the remaining ¾ cup of Parmesan cheese, and cover with aluminum foil. Bake for 10 minutes. Remove the foil and bake for an additional 5 minutes, or until bubbly and cheese is golden and melted. Serve warm, garnished with chopped parsley.

INGREDIENT TIP: Reserve the seeds in step 1 and roast them for a quick and nutritious keto-friendly snack. Remove the stringy membrane from the seeds, rinse, and drain them in a colander. Roast on a baking sheet lined with parchment paper at 400°F until dried and just golden, 10 to 12 minutes. Allow the seeds to cool and toss with 1 tablespoon of olive oil, ½ teaspoon of salt, and ½ teaspoon of cinnamon (optional) for a sweet and savory snack.

MACRONUTRIENTS: 74% Fat, 20% Protein, 6% Carbs

PER SERVING: Calories: 565; Total Fat: 47g; Saturated Fat: 15g; Protein: 26g; Total Carbs: 10g; Fiber: 1g; Net Carbs: 9g

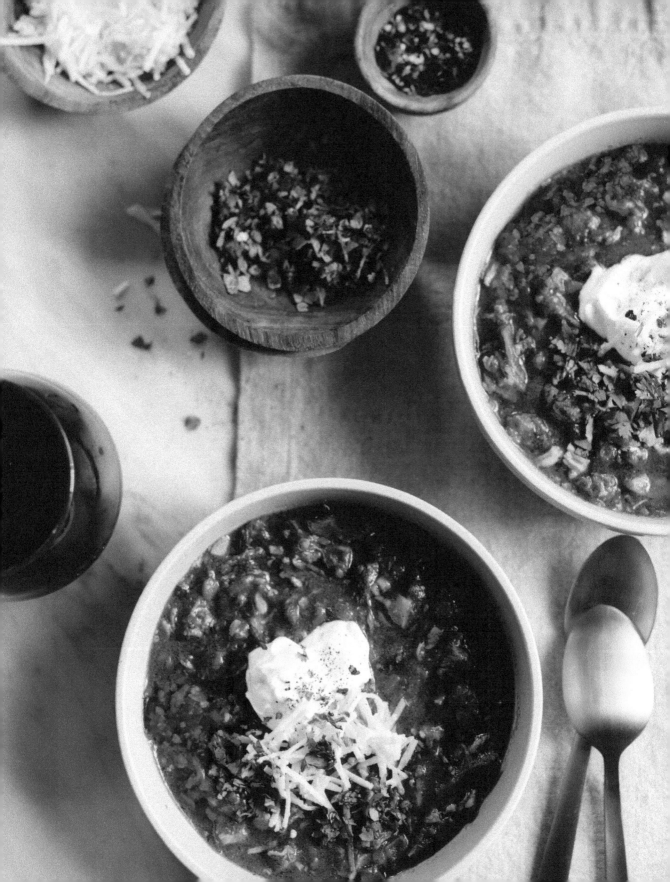

Meat

Eggplant Parmesan Lasagna

SERVES 8

Prep Time: 40 minutes / **Cook Time:** 1 hour

Freezer-Friendly

Who doesn't love lasagna? You don't have to say goodbye to this comfort food classic just because you're looking out for your health and following a ketogenic diet. With no pasta and all the flavor, this recipe is an adaptation of two classic favorites in one tasty, low-carb dish. It takes a little time to prepare, but it's well worth the effort.

½ cup extra-virgin olive oil, divided

2 eggs, beaten

2 teaspoons salt, divided

1 cup shredded Parmesan cheese, divided

2½ cups mozzarella cheese, divided

2 small eggplants, unpeeled, trimmed and cut into ¼-inch rounds

1 pound ground beef, preferably grass-fed

2 cups whole-milk ricotta cheese

2 teaspoons dried basil or oregano

¼ teaspoon freshly ground black pepper

3 cups Basic Marinara (page 125)

1. Preheat the oven to 425°F. Line a baking sheet with aluminum foil and coat with 2 tablespoons of olive oil.

2. In a small, shallow bowl, combine the beaten eggs and 1 teaspoon of salt. In a second bowl, combine ½ cup of Parmesan cheese and ½ cup of mozzarella cheese.

3. One at a time, dredge each eggplant round first in the egg mixture and then in the cheese mixture, coating each side. Place the coated eggplant rounds on the prepared baking sheet and drizzle with 2 tablespoons of olive oil. Bake until golden brown and eggplant is softened, 18 to 20 minutes.

4. While the eggplant bakes, prepare the filling. Heat 2 tablespoons of olive oil in a large skillet over medium heat. Add the ground beef and cook, breaking it apart, until browned and cooked through, 5 to 6 minutes. Do not drain.

5. To the skillet with the beef, stir in the ricotta cheese, basil, remaining 1 teaspoon of salt, and the pepper. Remove from the heat and set aside.

6. In a medium bowl, combine the marinara sauce with the remaining 2 tablespoons of olive oil and whisk until smooth. In a small bowl, combine the remaining 2 cups of mozzarella and ½ cup of Parmesan.

7. Once the eggplant is cooked, assemble the lasagna. Spoon one-third of the sauce mixture into a 9-by-13-inch glass baking dish and spread evenly to coat the bottom. Place half of the eggplant rounds in one layer to fully cover the sauce. Add half of the beef and ricotta mixture on top of the eggplant, spreading evenly. Top with half of the cheese mixture. Repeat another layer with sauce, eggplant, beef and ricotta, and cheese, topping with the final third of the sauce mixture.

8. Bake until the cheese is bubbly and melted, 30 to 35 minutes. Turn the broiler to low and broil until the top is golden brown, about 5 minutes.

9. Remove from the oven and allow to cool slightly before slicing.

INGREDIENT TIP: If you don't have any Basic Marinara Sauce on hand, you can substitute 2¾ cups of no-sugar-added jarred marinara sauce plus ½ cup of olive oil. Look for brands that have less than 5g of sugar per ½ cup serving.

MACRONUTRIENTS: 69% Fat, 20% Protein, 11% Carbs

PER SERVING: Calories: 662; Total Fat: 51g; Saturated Fat: 19g; Protein: 33g; Total Carbs: 17g; Fiber: 6g; Net Carbs: 11g

Cheesy Southwestern Meat Loaf

SERVES 8

Prep Time: 30 minutes, plus 10 minutes to rest

Cook Time: 1 hour

Protein Power

Many meat loaf recipes include bread crumbs and a sugary ketchup sauce. This one uses zucchini for moisture, texture, and nutrition, as well as less tomato sauce to reduce sugars. Fresh chorizo, a spiced pork sausage, is common in Latin American cuisine; just don't use dry chorizo, which is more like salami in texture. I find it in my local grocery store ground or in casings, but if you can't find it, you can substitute hot Italian sausage.

½ cup avocado or extra-virgin olive oil, divided

2 cups shredded (not spiralized) zucchini, from 2 small or 1 large zucchini

1½ teaspoons salt, divided

1 pound ground beef, preferably grass-fed

1 pound ground pork chorizo

½ cup chopped cilantro

¼ cup chopped scallions, green and white parts

1 large egg, beaten

1 tablespoon chopped chipotle pepper with adobo sauce (see ingredient tip)

1 teaspoon garlic powder

¼ cup almond flour

2 cups shredded Mexican cheese blend or cheddar cheese, divided

1 tablespoon tomato paste (no sugar added)

1. Preheat the oven to 375°F. Coat a loaf pan with 2 tablespoons of avocado oil.

2. Line a colander with a layer of paper towels and add the shredded zucchini. Sprinkle with ½ teaspoon of salt, tossing to coat. Let sit for 10 minutes, then press down with another layer of paper towels to release some of the excess moisture.

3. While the zucchini drains, in a large bowl, combine the ground beef, chorizo, cilantro, scallions, ¼ cup of oil, egg, chipotle with adobo, garlic powder, and remaining 1 teaspoon of salt. Mix well with a fork.

4. Add the almond flour to the drained zucchini and toss to coat. Add the zucchini to the meat mixture and mix until well combined. Add half of the mixture to the prepared pan and spread evenly. Top with 1 cup of shredded cheese, spreading evenly. Top with the remaining half of the mixture and spread evenly.

5. In a small bowl, whisk together the tomato paste and remaining 2 tablespoons of oil and spread evenly on top of the meat mixture. Sprinkle with the remaining 1 cup of cheese. Bake for 50 to 55 minutes, or until cooked through. Let sit for 10 minutes before cutting.

INGREDIENT TIP: Chipotle peppers in adobo are sold in a 4- to 6-ounce can in the Mexican food aisle. A little goes a long way, but you can store the rest in a glass container, covered in the refrigerator for up to 2 weeks, or in the freezer for up to 3 months (and scrape off what you need for future recipes). You can also use chili powder for a less spicy option.

MACRONUTRIENTS: 75% Fat, 22% Protein, 3% Carbs

PER SERVING: Calories: 623; Total Fat: 53g; Saturated Fat: 18g; Protein: 33g; Total Carbs: 4g; Fiber: 1g; Net Carbs: 3g

Shepherd's Pie

SERVES 6   *Freezer-Friendly*
Prep Time: 15 minutes / **Cook Time:** 70 minutes

A spin-off of a traditional Irish meal and a favorite among my clients, this cozy recipe comes together with very little hands-on time. It's also freezer-friendly, so I suggest doubling the recipe to make a second pie to freeze. To serve later, allow to thaw completely in the refrigerator overnight, and bake at 375°F for 20 to 25 minutes or until heated through.

4 tablespoons extra-virgin olive oil, divided

2 cups cauliflower florets (from about half a head of cauliflower)

2 tablespoons unsalted butter

½ cup heavy cream

1 cup shredded cheddar cheese

2 teaspoons salt, divided

2 teaspoons dried thyme, divided

½ teaspoon freshly ground black pepper, divided

1 pound ground beef, preferably grass-fed

½ small yellow onion, diced

1 cup chopped cabbage

1 carrot, peeled and diced

2 ribs celery, diced

4 ounces mushrooms, sliced

4 cloves garlic, minced

1 (14½-ounce) can diced tomatoes, with juices

2 tablespoons tomato paste

½ cup beef stock

8 ounces cream cheese, room temperature

1. Heat the oven to 375°F.

2. Heat 2 tablespoons of olive oil in a medium saucepan over medium-low heat. Add the cauliflower and sauté until just tender, 6 to 8 minutes. Add the butter and heavy cream, cover, reduce heat to low, and cook until cauliflower is very tender, another 6 to 8 minutes. Remove from the heat and allow to cool slightly.

3. Add the cheese, 1 teaspoon of salt, 1 teaspoon of thyme, and ¼ teaspoon of pepper to the cauliflower. Using an immersion blender or hand mixer, puree until very smooth. Set aside.

4. In a large saucepan or skillet, heat the remaining 2 tablespoons of olive oil over medium heat. Add the ground beef and sauté for 5 minutes, breaking apart the meat. Add the onion, cabbage, carrot, celery, and mushrooms and sauté for another 5 to 6 minutes, or until the vegetables are just tender and the meat is browned. Add the garlic, remaining 1 teaspoon of salt, remaining 1 teaspoon of thyme, and remaining ¼ teaspoon of pepper and sauté, stirring, for another 30 seconds.

5. Stir in the tomatoes with their juices and the tomato paste. Bring to a simmer, reduce heat to low, cover, and simmer for 8 to 10 minutes, or until the vegetables are very tender and sauce has thickened.

6. In a small microwave-safe bowl, combine the stock and cream cheese and microwave on high for 1 minute or until cheese is melted. Whisk until creamy.

7. Add the cream cheese mixture to the meat and vegetables and stir to combine well. Place the mixture in an 8-inch square glass baking dish or pie pan. Spread the pureed cauliflower over the meat mixture and bake until golden, 25 to 30 minutes.

MACRONUTRIENTS: 76% Fat, 16% Protein, 8% Carbs

PER SERVING: Calories: 868; Total Fat: 74g; Saturated Fat: 35g; Protein: 37g; Total Carbs: 18g; Fiber: 5g; Net Carbs: 13g

Beef and Broccoli Foil Packs

SERVES 4

Prep Time: 10 minutes, plus 1 hour to marinate
Cook Time: 10 minutes

Freezer-Friendly

One of my favorite prep-in-advance meals, these foil packs are easy to prepare and freeze beautifully. To reheat, simply place a thawed foil pack on a hot grill, and dinner is ready in a flash. Alternatively, these can be baked in the oven at 400°F for 10 to 12 minutes.

¼ cup beef stock

¼ cup low-sodium soy sauce

¼ cup sesame oil

¼ cup plus 2 tablespoons extra-virgin olive oil, divided

4 cloves garlic, minced

2 tablespoons chopped fresh ginger

1 pound flank steak, sliced against the grain into ¼-inch strips

2 cups broccoli florets, cut into bite-size pieces

¼ cup minced scallion, green and white parts

2 tablespoons sesame seeds

1. In a small bowl, whisk together the stock, soy sauce, sesame oil, ¼ cup of olive oil, the garlic, and ginger. Pour half of the mixture into a large zip-top plastic bag and add the steak slices. Marinate in the refrigerator for at least 1 hour, up to 24 hours.

2. Heat the remaining 2 tablespoons of olive oil in a large skillet over high heat. Remove the steak from the marinade and discard the marinade. Sear the steak for 2 to 3 minutes, until just browned on each side, but not cooked through.

3. Lay four 8-inch squares of aluminum foil on the counter. Place ½ cup of broccoli and a quarter of the seared steak in the middle of each piece of foil. Pour a quarter of the remaining soy sauce mixture over each steak and broccoli pile, garnish with the scallions and sesame seeds, and cover with a second 8-inch foil square. Fold the foil up to about 1 inch from the mixture on each side. Fold in each corner once to secure and seal the foil pack.

4. Preheat the grill on medium-high heat. Place the prepared foil packs in a single layer on the grill and grill for 6 to 8 minutes, or until the steak is cooked through and the broccoli is fork-tender.

PREP TIP: If preparing these in a larger batch to freeze for later, follow steps 1 through 3 and place the packs on a baking sheet in the freezer for 2 hours, or until the liquid is frozen. Transfer the packs to a freezer-safe zip-top bag and store for later use.

MACRONUTRIENTS: 74% Fat, 21% Protein, 5% Carbs

PER SERVING: Calories: 547; Total Fat: 46g; Saturated Fat: 9g; Protein: 28g; Total Carbs: 7g; Fiber: 2g; Net Carbs: 5g

Weeknight Chili

SERVES 6

Prep Time: 10 minutes / **Cook Time:** 35 minutes

Protein Power

Chili doesn't have to include carb-heavy beans to be tasty, filling, and comforting. This version uses a combination of beef and pork, but feel free to substitute veal, venison, or all beef for the pork. Add extra cayenne or red pepper flakes for added heat and a sprinkle of cilantro for some freshness.

¼ cup extra-virgin olive oil

1 small yellow onion, diced

1 green bell pepper, diced

1 pound ground beef, preferably grass-fed

½ pound ground Italian sausage (hot or sweet)

1 tablespoon chili powder

2 teaspoons ground cumin

1½ teaspoons salt

6 cloves garlic, minced

1 (14½-ounce) can diced tomatoes, with juices

1 (6-ounce) can tomato paste

2 cups water

2 ripe avocados, pitted, peeled, and chopped

1 cup sour cream

1. Heat the olive oil in a large pot over medium heat. Add the onion and bell pepper and sauté for 5 minutes, or until just tender.

2. Add the ground beef and sausage and cook until meat is browned, 5 to 6 minutes, stirring to break into small pieces. Add the chili powder, cumin, salt, and garlic and sauté, stirring frequently, for 1 minute, until fragrant.

3. Add the tomatoes and their juices, tomato paste, and water, stirring to combine well. Bring the mixture to a boil, reduce heat to low, cover, and simmer for 15 to 20 minutes, stirring occasionally. Add additional water for a thinner chili if desired.

4. Serve hot, garnished with chopped avocado and sour cream.

MACRONUTRIENTS: 72% Fat, 16% Protein, 11% Carbs

PER SERVING: Calories: 591; Total Fat: 49g; Saturated Fat: 15g; Protein: 25g; Total Carbs: 18g; Fiber: 8g; Net Carbs: 10g

Slow Cooker Herb-and-Garlic Short Rib Stew

SERVES 4

Prep Time: 10 minutes / **Cook Time:** 4 to 6 hours

Protein Power

Short ribs are the ultimate in keto luxury. Full of flavor and fat, they are an ideal option for a rich, crowd-pleasing meal. Feel free to substitute the wine with all beef stock. For a real treat, serve with Keto Biscuits (in the Biscuit-Topped Chicken Pot Pie recipe, page 92) or Microwave Keto Bread (page 120).

1 pound boneless beef
   short ribs

1 teaspoon salt

½ teaspoon garlic powder

¼ teaspoon freshly ground
   black pepper

4 tablespoons extra-virgin
   olive oil, divided

½ small yellow onion, diced

1 carrot, peeled and diced

2 ribs celery, diced

4 ounces sliced mushrooms

6 cloves garlic, minced

2 teaspoons dried thyme

2 teaspoons dried rosemary
   (or 2 tablespoons fresh)

1 teaspoon dried oregano

3 cups beef stock

1 (14½-ounce) can diced
   tomatoes, with juices

½ cup dry red wine (such
   as merlot)

1. Season the short ribs with the salt, garlic powder, and pepper.

2. Heat 2 tablespoons of olive oil in a large skillet over high heat. Add the short ribs and brown until dark in color, 2 to 3 minutes per side. Transfer to the bowl of a slow cooker.

3. Add the remaining 2 tablespoons of olive oil to the skillet and reduce heat to medium. Add the onion, carrot, celery, and mushrooms and sauté until just tender but not fully cooked, 3 to 4 minutes. Add the garlic and sauté, stirring, for an additional 30 seconds. Transfer the contents of the skillet to the slow cooker with the ribs.

4. Add the thyme, rosemary, oregano, stock, tomatoes with their juices, and wine, and cook on low for 4 to 6 hours, or until meat is very tender.

5. Remove the ribs from the stew and shred using two forks. Return the shredded meat to the stew and stir to combine well. Serve warm.

VARIATION TIP: To make this recipe on the stovetop, brown the short ribs and vegetables as directed in steps 2 and 3 in a large Dutch oven or deep skillet. Add the herbs and liquid, cover, and transfer to an oven heated to 350°F. Cook for 1½ to 2 hours or until ribs are very tender. Finish with step 5.

MACRONUTRIENTS: 73% Fat, 18% Protein, 10% Carbs

PER SERVING: Calories: 549; Total Fat: 43g; Saturated Fat: 12g; Protein: 24g; Total Carbs: 14g; Fiber: 5g; Net Carbs: 9g

Steak with Blue Cheese Butter

SERVES 4

Prep Time: 5 minutes, plus 35 minutes to rest
Cook Time: 10 minutes

Protein Power

Skillet roasting is hands-down the easiest indoor steak cooking method. Steak alone is high in protein-to-fat ratios, but the blue cheese butter helps keep those ratios keto-friendly in this restaurant-worthy dish. You can double or quadruple this blue cheese butter recipe to have on hand for other uses—it will keep in the refrigerator for up to 1 week or the freezer for up to 3 months.

4 (4-ounce) filet mignon or New York strip steaks

1 teaspoon salt

1 teaspoon garlic powder, divided

¼ teaspoon freshly ground black pepper

¼ cup unsalted butter, room temperature

¼ cup crumbled blue cheese

½ teaspoon dried thyme

2 tablespoons extra-virgin olive oil

1. Preheat the oven to 450°F. Rub the steaks with the salt, ½ teaspoon of garlic powder, and the pepper. Let sit at room temperature for 15 to 30 minutes.

2. To make the blue cheese butter, in a small bowl, combine the butter, blue cheese, remaining ½ teaspoon of garlic powder, and thyme and whisk until well combined and smooth. Set aside.

3. Heat the olive oil in a large, oven-proof skillet over high heat. When the oil is very hot, add the steaks and sear for 1 minute on each side. Transfer the skillet to the oven and roast to desired doneness. For 1-inch-thick steaks, it will take 3 to 6 minutes for rare (130 to 135°F), 6 to 8 minutes for medium-rare (140 to 155°F), and 8 to 10 minutes for well-done (150 to 155°F). For 1½-inch-thick steaks, cook 4 to 6 minutes for rare and 8 to 10 minutes for well-done.

4. Remove the steaks from the skillet and place each on a separate plate. Top each with 2 tablespoons of blue cheese butter and allow the steak to rest and butter to melt for 5 minutes before serving.

MACRONUTRIENTS: 75% Fat, 24% Protein, 1% Carbs

PER SERVING: Calories: 437; Total Fat: 37g; Saturated Fat: 16g; Protein: 25g; Total Carbs: 1g; Fiber: 0g; Net Carbs: 1g

Lamb Kebabs with Mint and Pistachio Pesto

SERVES 4

Prep Time: 15 minutes, plus 1 hour to marinate

Cook Time: 15 minutes

Brain Health

Lamb has a higher fat-to-protein ratio, making it an ideal protein for a ketogenic diet and great for producing brain-boosting ketone power. This inventive recipe takes the classic mint and lamb pairing to a keto-friendly level. Serve it over salad or with Cauliflower Fried Rice (page 121).

1½ cups fresh mint leaves

¼ cup shelled pistachios

2 cloves garlic, chopped

Zest and juice of 1 orange

¼ cup sesame oil

1 teaspoon salt

¼ teaspoon freshly ground black pepper

¼ cup extra-virgin olive oil

½ cup apple cider vinegar

1 pound boneless leg of lamb, cut into 1-inch cubes

1. Combine the mint, pistachios, and garlic in the bowl of a food processor or blender and process until very finely chopped. Add the orange zest and juice, sesame oil, salt, and pepper, and pulse until smooth. With the processor running, stream in the olive oil until smooth.

2. Place ¼ cup of the mint pesto in a small bowl, add the vinegar, and whisk to form a marinade. Place the lamb cubes in the marinade and toss to coat. Cover and refrigerate for at least 1 hour, up to 24 hours.

3. While the lamb is marinating, soak four wooden skewers in water for 30 to 60 minutes. Preheat the oven to 450°F.

4. Thread the lamb cubes onto the soaked skewers, dividing evenly among the four. Place the skewers on a broiler pan or rimmed baking sheet lined with foil.

5. Cook until browned and cooked through, 12 to 15 minutes, flipping halfway through cooking time.

6. Serve the skewers drizzled with the remaining mint pesto.

VARIATION TIP: These kebabs are fabulous prepared on the grill. In step 4, preheat the grill to medium-high heat and grill for 4 to 5 minutes per side, or until cooked through.

MACRONUTRIENTS: 79% Fat, 15% Protein, 6% Carbs

PER SERVING: Calories: 592; Total Fat: 52g; Saturated Fat: 17g; Protein: 22g; Total Carbs: 5g; Fiber: 1g; Net Carbs: 4g

Sausage Stuffing

SERVES 4 as a main or 8 as a side

Prep Time: 15 minutes, plus 10 minutes to rest

Cook Time: 45 minutes

Freezer-Friendly

Great for Thanksgiving or any occasion, this veggie-loaded casserole is full of warm fall flavors. It uses crispy cauliflower in place of the bread and adds crumbled sausage for protein, making it a filling side or complete one-dish meal.

4 cups cauliflower florets (about half of a head), broken or chopped into ½-inch pieces

½ cup extra-virgin olive oil, divided

1 teaspoon salt, divided

8 ounces bulk pork sausage (Italian mild or unsweetened breakfast)

½ small onion, diced small

4 ribs celery, diced small

¼ cup chopped carrot (about 1 small carrot)

4 ounces chopped mushrooms

1 tablespoon fresh sage, finely chopped (or 2 teaspoons dried)

1 teaspoon dried thyme

¼ teaspoon freshly ground black pepper

4 cloves garlic, minced

1 cup chicken or vegetable stock

¼ cup dry white wine (or additional stock)

2 tablespoons fresh parsley, chopped

1. Preheat the oven to 425°F and line a rimmed baking sheet with aluminum foil.

2. In a large bowl, toss the cauliflower with ¼ cup of olive oil and ½ teaspoon of salt. Spread the cauliflower in a single layer on the prepared baking sheet, reserving the bowl.

3. Cook the cauliflower until golden brown and crispy but not soft, 10 to 12 minutes. Remove from the oven, reduce heat to 375°F, and allow the cauliflower to cool slightly before transferring back to the reserved bowl.

4. Heat the remaining ¼ cup of olive oil in a large skillet over medium-high heat. Add the sausage and brown for 10 minutes, breaking it into small pieces. Do not drain the rendered fat.

5. To the skillet with the sausage, add the onion, celery, carrot, mushrooms, sage, thyme, remaining ½ teaspoon of salt, and pepper and sauté until the vegetables begin to soften, 5 to 7 minutes. Add the garlic and sauté, stirring, for another 30 seconds.

6. Add the stock and white wine, increase heat to high, and sauté, continuously stirring, until half the liquid evaporates.

7. Transfer the sausage-and-vegetable mixture to the bowl with the cauliflower and stir in the parsley. Transfer the mixture to an 8-inch square glass baking dish.

8. Bake uncovered until the top is browned and crispy, 15 to 20 minutes. Allow to rest for 10 minutes before serving.

MAKE-AHEAD TIP: The stuffing can be prepped ahead up to step 8 and either kept in the refrigerator up to 24 hours or frozen for up to 3 months. Thaw before baking at 375°F uncovered.

MACRONUTRIENTS: 83% Fat, 10% Protein, 7% Carbs

PER SERVING: Calories: 496; Total Fat: 45g; Saturated Fat: 10g; Protein: 12g; Total Carbs: 10g; Fiber: 3g; Net Carbs: 7g

Slow Cooker Swedish Meatballs

SERVES 8 (about 4 meatballs per serving)

Prep Time: 20 minutes / **Cook Time:** 4 hours

Protein Power

Contrary to popular belief, Swedish meatballs did not originate in Sweden at all, but come from Turkish cuisine, which is why they include spices like nutmeg and allspice. This recipe makes this rich and flavorful dish even easier and perfect for entertaining by adapting it for the slow cooker. I've included ground ginger in the spice mixture, which I think really adds to the flavor profile. Feel free to omit it if you're a traditionalist!

1 pound ground Italian
   pork sausage

1 pound ground beef,
   preferably grass-fed

½ small yellow
   onion, minced

¼ cup almond flour

1 large egg, beaten

3 teaspoons Worcestershire
   sauce, divided

2 teaspoons salt, divided

1 teaspoon ground allspice

½ teaspoon ground nutmeg

½ teaspoon ground ginger

½ teaspoon freshly ground
   black pepper, divided

1½ cups beef stock or broth

1 cup heavy cream

1 tablespoon Dijon mustard

4 ounces cream cheese,
   room temperature

1 cup sour cream, room
   temperature

1. In a large bowl, combine the pork, beef, onion, almond flour, egg, 1 teaspoon of Worcestershire, 1 teaspoon of salt, the allspice, nutmeg, ginger, and ¼ teaspoon of pepper and mix well with a fork.

2. Form the meat mixture into small 1-inch meatballs, and place on a baking sheet or cutting board.

3. In the bowl of a 5- or 6-quart slow cooker, whisk together the stock, heavy cream, mustard, remaining 2 teaspoons of Worcestershire sauce, remaining 1 teaspoon of salt, and remaining ¼ teaspoon of pepper until smooth and creamy. Place the meatballs in the sauce, trying to not overcrowd. Set the slow cooker to low and cook for 4 hours.

4. After 4 hours of cooking, whisk together the cream cheese and sour cream and add to the warm mixture, gently stirring to incorporate well.

5. Serve the meatballs in their sauce with toothpicks, or over spiralized zucchini for a complete meal. Leftover meatballs and sauce can be frozen for up to 3 months.

VARIATION TIP: These meatballs can also be cooked on the stove top. Follow steps 1 and 2 to prepare the meatballs. Heat the sauce ingredients in step 3 in a large saucepan over medium-high heat until nearly simmering. Reduce heat to low, add the meatballs, cover, and cook until cooked through, 20 to 25 minutes. Place the cream cheese and sour cream in a small bowl. Spoon out ½ cup of the meatball cooking liquid and whisk into the cream cheese mixture until smooth. Stir into the pot with the meatballs until well combined.

MACRONUTRIENTS: 80% Fat, 17% Protein, 3% Carbs

PER SERVING: Calories: 544; Total Fat: 49g; Saturated Fat: 23g; Protein: 23g; Total Carbs: 5g; Fiber: 1g; Net Carbs: 4g

Crispy Baked Pork Chops with Mushroom Gravy

SERVES 4

Prep Time: 10 minutes / **Cook Time:** 25 minutes

Protein Power

This recipe is a throwback to my mom's go-to weekday meal, made with Shake 'n Bake and cream of mushroom soup. Fast-forward 30 years, and I made a recipe filled with good fats, no fillers, and loaded with quality protein. Delicious and still perfect for a busy weekday.

4 tablespoons extra-virgin olive oil, divided

½ cup almond flour

2 teaspoons dried sage, divided

1½ teaspoons salt, divided

½ teaspoon freshly ground black pepper, divided

1 large egg

¼ cup flax meal

¼ cup walnuts, very finely chopped

4 (4-ounce) boneless pork chops

1 tablespoon unsalted butter

4 ounces chopped mushrooms

2 cloves garlic, minced

1 teaspoon dried thyme

8 ounces cream cheese, room temperature

½ cup heavy cream

¼ cup chicken stock

1. Preheat the oven to 400°F. Line a baking sheet with aluminum foil and coat with 1 tablespoon of olive oil.

2. In a small, shallow bowl, combine the almond flour, 1 teaspoon of sage, ½ teaspoon of salt, and ¼ teaspoon of pepper. In a second small bowl, whisk the egg. In a third small bowl, stir together the flax meal and walnuts.

3. One at a time, dredge each pork chop first in the flour mixture, then in the egg, then in the flax-and-walnut mixture to fully coat all sides. Place on the prepared baking sheet and drizzle the pork chops evenly with 1 tablespoon of olive oil.

4. Bake until cooked through and golden brown, 18 to 25 minutes, depending on the thickness of the pork.

5. While the pork is baking, prepare the gravy. Heat the remaining 2 tablespoons of olive oil and the butter in a medium saucepan over medium heat. Add the mushrooms and sauté until very tender, 4 to 6 minutes. Add the garlic, remaining 1 teaspoon of sage and 1 teaspoon of salt, thyme, and remaining ¼ teaspoon of pepper, and sauté for an additional 30 seconds.

6. Add the cream cheese to the mushrooms, reduce heat to low, and stir until melted and creamy, 2 to 3 minutes. Whisk in the cream and stock until smooth. Cook over low heat, whisking frequently, until the mixture is thick and creamy, another 3 to 4 minutes.

7. Serve each pork chop covered with a quarter of the mushroom gravy.

MACRONUTRIENTS: 77% Fat, 18% Protein, 5% Carbs

PER SERVING: Calories: 799; Total Fat: 69g; Saturated Fat: 25g; Protein: 36g; Total Carbs: 11g; Fiber: 4g; Net Carbs: 7g

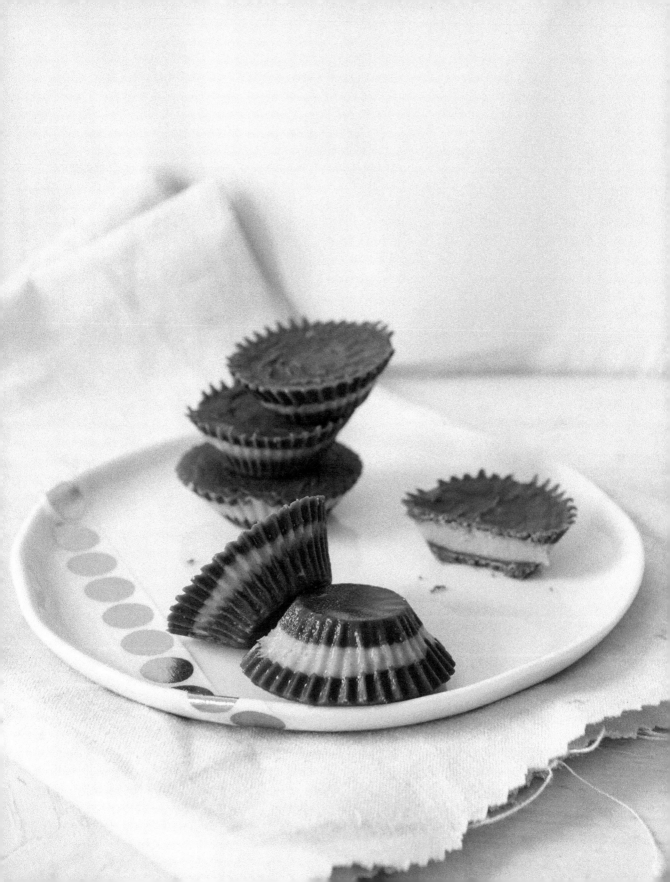

CHAPTER EIGHT

Staples, Broths, Sauces & Dressings

Microwave Keto Bread

MAKES 1 roll or 2 thin slices for a sandwich

Prep Time: 5 minutes / **Cook Time:** 90 seconds

Freezer-Friendly

Ready in a flash and used to accompany many of the recipes in this book, this recipe is a go-to when you just need a bread fix. Use as a roll to accompany soups or stews, or slice and toast for a keto-friendly morning avocado toast. Add caraway seeds to make a version reminiscent of rye bread.

1 large egg

3 tablespoons almond flour

1 tablespoon extra-virgin olive oil

¼ teaspoon baking powder

⅛ teaspoon salt

1. In a microwave-safe ramekin, small bowl, or mug, beat the egg. Add the almond flour, olive oil, baking powder, and salt and mix well with a fork.

2. Microwave on high for 90 seconds.

3. Slide a knife around the edges of the ramekin and flip to remove the bread.

4. Slice the bread in half with a serrated knife if you want to use it to make a sandwich.

VARIATION TIP: This bread can also be baked in a 375°F oven for 10 minutes.

MACRONUTRIENTS: 81% Fat, 14% Protein, 5% Carbs

PER SERVING: Calories: 264; Total Fat: 24g; Saturated Fat: 4g; Protein: 9g; Total Carbs: 4g; Fiber: 2g; Net Carbs: 2g

Cauliflower Fried Rice

SERVES 6 to 8
Prep Time: 15 minutes / **Cook Time:** 10 minutes

Reduces Inflammation

Cauliflower has become almost the mascot for a low-carb diet, and you'll find it substituted for grains or potatoes in many ketogenic recipes. Making your own riced cauliflower is easy and inexpensive, and preserves the texture. Be sure to fry it in a large, shallow skillet. Using a smaller, deeper pan will steam the cauliflower and make it mushy. This recipe is meant to serve as the base for many dishes, or feel free to add extra chopped veggies such as red peppers, mushrooms, onions, and celery, or cooked shrimp, chicken, tofu, or pork to make it a complete and really delicious meal.

1 small head cauliflower, bottom stem, leaves, and core removed, and broken into florets
1 large egg, beaten
1 tablespoon sesame oil
1 tablespoon soy sauce
3 tablespoons coconut oil
2 garlic cloves, minced

1. Place the cauliflower florets in a food processor and pulse several times, until the cauliflower is the consistency of rice or couscous.

2. Whisk together the egg, sesame oil, and soy sauce.

3. In a large skillet, heat the coconut oil over medium-high heat. Add the riced cauliflower and sauté, stirring constantly with a spatula, for 3 to 4 minutes, or until starting to brown. Add the garlic and sauté, stirring, for an additional 30 seconds.

4. Add the egg mixture, again stirring constantly, until all the moisture has evaporated and the egg is cooked through, another 2 to 3 minutes. Remove from the heat and serve immediately.

VARIATION TIP: This recipe mimics restaurant fried rice, but feel free to vary the spices and flavors to complement any main dish. You can replace the coconut and sesame oil for olive oil, substitute Worcestershire sauce for the soy sauce, and add chopped fresh herbs such as parsley, cilantro, or rosemary.

MACRONUTRIENTS: 83% Fat, 8% Protein, 9% Carbs

PER SERVING: Calories: 104; Total Fat: 10g; Saturated Fat: 7g; Protein: 2g; Total Carbs: 3g; Fiber: 1g; Net Carbs: 2g

Cashew Hummus

MAKES about 1 cup (2 tablespoons per serving)
Prep Time: 5 minutes, plus 12 hours to soak

Reduces Inflammation

Hummus is a part of many healthy diets; however, it's very high in carbohydrates, making it unfriendly on a ketogenic diet as well as a potential inflammation trigger for many. This recipe use anti-inflammatory nuts, seeds, and oil without the legumes that can cause issues for many people. The cashews will need to be soaked in water overnight. Be sure not to skip this step to ensure a smooth consistency.

1 cup raw cashews

2 small cloves garlic, peeled

3 tablespoons tahini

1 tablespoon lemon juice

1 teaspoon salt

½ teaspoon smoked paprika

¼ cup extra-virgin olive oil

1. Place the cashews in a medium bowl and cover with cold water. Cover the bowl and soak in the refrigerator overnight or up to 24 hours.

2. Drain the water from the cashews and place them in the bowl of a food processor. Add the garlic and tahini and process until smooth but thick. Add the lemon juice, salt, and paprika and pulse until well combined.

3. With the processor running, stream in the olive oil and process until very smooth and silky but not runny. Serve with raw veggies for dipping, such as celery, cucumber, bell pepper, or broccoli. Leftover hummus can be stored in a sealed container in the refrigerator for up to 4 days.

INGREDIENT TIP: Tahini, or ground sesame seed paste, can be found in the aisle with the nut butters or ethnic foods in most grocery stores. It is the classic flavor in traditional hummus, but you can substitute an additional ¼ cup of cashews, soaked in water overnight, for the same consistency but without the flavor.

MACRONUTRIENTS: 77% Fat, 8% Protein, 15% Carbs

PER SERVING: Calories: 199; Total Fat: 18g; Saturated Fat: 3g; Protein: 4g; Total Carbs: 7g; Fiber: 1g; Net Carbs: 6g

Any-Herb Pesto

MAKES about 1 cup (2 tablespoons per serving)
Prep Time: 5 minutes

Brain Health

Pesto may sound fancy, but it's really just a flavorful combination of herbs, garlic, sometimes cheese and nuts, and heart-healthy, anti-inflammatory olive oil. This recipe puts a spin on traditional basil pesto with the addition of arugula, but feel free to mix up the flavors with whatever you may have in the refrigerator. Not only is this a great way to add intense flavor to your meal, but it also makes leaner cuts of meat, such as chicken breast or seafood, fit into the ketogenic diet.

4 cups packed baby
    arugula leaves
1 cup packed basil leaves
1 cup walnuts, chopped
½ cup shredded
    Parmesan cheese
2 small garlic cloves, peeled
    and smashed
½ teaspoon salt
¾ cup extra-virgin olive oil

1. In a food processor, pulse the arugula, basil, walnuts, cheese, and garlic until very finely chopped. Add the salt. With the processor running, stream in the olive oil until well blended and smooth.

2. Transfer the mixture to a glass container and store, tightly covered in the refrigerator, for up to 2 weeks.

VARIATION TIP: Traditional pesto uses basil, Parmesan, and pine nuts, but I love to use whatever herbs or greens I have on hand—this enables me to come up with new flavors to complement meals. Combinations to try: parsley and almonds; cilantro, red pepper flakes, and pumpkin seeds; or mint, sesame oil, and peanuts.

MACRONUTRIENTS: 90% Fat, 5% Protein, 5% Carbs

PER SERVING: Calories: 305; Total Fat: 32g; Saturated Fat: 5g; Protein: 4g; Total Carbs: 4g; Fiber: 1g; Net Carbs: 3g

Keto Peanut Butter Cups

MAKES 16

Prep Time: 5 minutes, plus 2½ hours to chill
Cook Time: 2 minutes

Freezer-Friendly

These easy keto treats will satisfy a snack or sweet craving in an instant. I encourage my patients to keep a batch on hand for when that urge strikes. Easy to make and devoid of artificial fillers, they are the ultimate convenient snack.

½ cup cacao butter or coconut oil

¼ cup unsweetened cocoa powder

2 to 4 teaspoons sugar-free sweetener of choice (optional)

½ teaspoon cinnamon (optional)

½ teaspoon salt

½ cup unsweetened creamy peanut butter or almond butter

1. Line a mini muffin tin with 16 liners.

2. Place the cacao butter and cocoa powder into a microwave-safe bowl and microwave on high for 30 to 45 seconds or until melted. Stir until creamy.

3. Whisk in the sweetener (if using), cinnamon (if using), and salt. Spoon half of the chocolate mixture into the 16 cups, spreading to cover the bottom of the liner. Reserve the other half of the chocolate mixture. Place the pan in the freezer for 10 minutes to set.

4. In a small, microwave-safe bowl, microwave the nut butter for 30 seconds, until soft, then spread on top of the chocolate in the cups. Freeze for 10 minutes.

5. Microwave the cacao butter mixture for an additional 30 seconds, just to soften it. Dollop the remaining chocolate on top of the nut butter.

6. Return the pan to the freezer and freeze until solid, about 2 hours. Once frozen, peanut butter cups can be transferred to a zip-top bag and stored in the refrigerator for up to 2 weeks or the freezer for up to 3 months.

VARIATION TIP: You can simply melt the cocoa powder, cacao butter, and peanut butter together, combine with the other ingredients, and pour it into lined mini or regular-size muffin tins.

MACRONUTRIENTS: 88% Fat, 6% Protein, 6% Carbs

PER SERVING: Calories: 111; Total Fat: 11g; Saturated Fat: 5g; Protein: 2g; Total Carbs: 2g; Fiber: 1g; Net Carbs: 1g

Basic Marinara

MAKES about 4 cups (½ cup per serving)
Prep Time: 15 minutes / **Cook Time:** 1 hour

Reduces Inflammation

While there are many lower-sugar marinara sauce brands available on the market now, they are often very pricey, making homemade options more appealing. Making your own sauce will save you money—plus, since you control the ingredients, you can also maximize the health benefits by including heart-health anti-inflammatory olive oil and fresh vegetables. This sauce is freezable, so feel free to double the recipe to make an extra jar for later.

2 tablespoons plus ¼ cup extra-virgin olive oil, divided

2 tablespoons unsalted butter

½ small onion, finely minced

2 ribs celery, finely minced

¼ cup minced carrot (about 1 small carrot)

4 cloves garlic, minced

1 teaspoon salt

¼ teaspoon freshly ground black pepper

1 (32-ounce) can crushed tomatoes, with juices

2 tablespoons balsamic vinegar

1 teaspoon dried oregano

1 teaspoon dried rosemary

½ to 1 teaspoon red pepper flakes (optional)

1. Heat 2 tablespoons of olive oil and the butter in a medium saucepan over medium heat. Add the onion, celery, and carrot and sauté until just starting to get tender, about 5 minutes. Add the garlic, salt, and pepper and sauté for an additional 30 seconds.

2. Whisk in the tomatoes and their juices, vinegar, remaining ¼ cup of olive oil, oregano, rosemary, and red pepper (if using). Bring to a simmer, cover, reduce heat to low, and simmer for 30 to 60 minutes to allow the flavors to blend. Serve warm. The sauce will keep, tightly covered in the refrigerator, for up to 1 week. Cooled sauce can be frozen for up to 3 months.

MACRONUTRIENTS: 82% Fat, 2% Protein, 16% Carbs

PER SERVING: Calories: 144; Total Fat: 13g; Saturated Fat: 3g; Protein: 1g; Total Carbs: 6g; Fiber: 3g; Net Carbs: 3g

Coconut-Curry Simmer Sauce

MAKES 2 cups
Prep Time: 5 minutes / **Cook Time:** 5 minutes

Reduces Inflammation

Inspired by my husband and his love for Pacific cuisine, this sauce is a wonderfully delicious and rich alternative for many bottled simmer sauces. It enables dinner to come together in a flash. Simply add the entire recipe to 2 pounds of chicken thighs, pork, or lamb; add to the slow cooker; and cook over low heat for 4 to 6 hours or until tender. Dinner done!

1 (14½-ounce) can full-fat
   coconut milk
Zest and juice of 1 lime
2 tablespoons curry powder
1 tablespoon soy sauce
1 teaspoon ground ginger
1 teaspoon garlic powder
½ to 1 teaspoon
   cayenne pepper

Whisk all the ingredients in a small saucepan over medium-high heat and bring just below a boil. Remove from heat and allow to cool to room temperature. The sauce will keep, tightly covered in the refrigerator, for up to 1 week.

MACRONUTRIENTS: 85% Fat, 5% Protein, 10% Carbs

PER SERVING (½ CUP): Calories: 221; Total Fat: 22g; Saturated Fat: 19g; Protein: 3g; Total Carbs: 7g; Fiber: 2g; Net Carbs: 5g

Versatile Tartar Sauce

MAKES about ½ cup (1 tablespoon per serving)
Prep Time: 5 minutes

Brain Health

This sauce is delicious on more than just seafood; I like it atop burgers or as the base of a simple tuna or salmon salad. Without any of the added sugars of restaurant or bottled brands, this still tastes delicious, and is also a great way to achieve your nutritional goals.

½ cup mayonnaise

2 tablespoons chopped dill pickles (not sweet)

1 tablespoon minced red onion

1 tablespoon freshly squeezed lemon juice

¼ teaspoon salt

¼ teaspoon freshly ground black pepper

In a small bowl or canning jar, combine all the ingredients and whisk well with a fork. Sauce will store covered in the refrigerator for up to 3 days.

VARIATION TIP: For a more sophisticated taste, substitute chopped capers for the pickles and add 1 tablespoon of finely chopped parsley. For a sauce with a kick, add 1 to 2 teaspoons of horseradish.

MACRONUTRIENTS: 98% Fat, 1% Protein, 1% Carbs

PER SERVING: Calories: 95; Total Fat: 10g; Saturated Fat: 2g; Protein: 0g; Total Carbs: 0g; Fiber: 0g; Net Carbs: 0g

Red Wine Vinaigrette

MAKES 1 cup (2 tablespoons per serving)
Prep Time: 5 minutes

Reduces Inflammation

Most store-bought vinaigrettes, even those without added sugar, are made with pro-inflammatory vegetable oils such as canola or soybean, which can exacerbate many health conditions over time. Making your own is so easy and provides the health benefit of reducing inflammation, and will save you money as well.

½ cup extra-virgin olive oil

½ cup red wine vinegar

1 tablespoon Dijon or stone-ground mustard

½ to 1 teaspoon dried herbs such as rosemary, basil, thyme, or oregano (optional)

½ teaspoon salt

¼ teaspoon freshly ground black pepper

In a small bowl or canning jar, combine all the ingredients and whisk or shake until well combined. The dressing will keep, tightly covered in the refrigerator, for up to 2 weeks. Be sure to bring it to room temperature and shake well before serving, as the oil and vinegar will naturally separate.

MACRONUTRIENTS: 99% Fat, <1% Protein, <1% Carbs

PER SERVING: Calories: 123; Total Fat: 14g; Saturated Fat: 2g; Protein: 0g; Total Carbs: 0g; Fiber: 0g; Net Carbs: 0g

Easiest Creamy Caesar Dressing

MAKES 1½ cups (2 tablespoons per serving)

Prep Time: 5 minutes

Brain Health

This simple and flavorful dressing will liven up any bowl of greens. Traditionally, Caesar dressing is served over torn romaine lettuce, but in my house, we enjoy this with everything from baby spinach or arugula to tuna or chicken salad.

1 cup mayonnaise

2 small garlic cloves, pressed with a garlic press (or 1 teaspoon garlic powder)

2 tablespoons freshly squeezed lemon juice, from 1 lemon

2 teaspoons Dijon mustard

1 teaspoon anchovy paste

1 teaspoon Worcestershire sauce

½ cup freshly grated Parmesan cheese

¼ teaspoon salt

¼ teaspoon freshly ground black pepper

1. In a canning jar or small bowl, combine the mayonnaise, garlic, lemon juice, mustard, anchovy paste, and Worcestershire and whisk well.

2. Add the cheese, salt, and pepper and whisk until well combined and smooth. The dressing will keep, tightly covered in the refrigerator, for up to 1 week. Shake or whisk again before serving.

INGREDIENT TIP: Anchovy paste is a staple in traditional Caesar dressing, but if you prefer, you can leave it out and substitute with an additional ½ teaspoon of salt and ½ teaspoon of Dijon.

MACRONUTRIENTS: 93% Fat, 4% Protein, 3% Carbs

PER SERVING: Calories: 145; Total Fat: 15g; Saturated Fat: 3g; Protein: 2g; Total Carbs: 1g; Fiber: 0g; Net Carbs: 1g

Tangy Citrus-Poppyseed Dressing

MAKES about 1 cup (2 tablespoons per serving)

Prep Time: 5 minutes

Bone Health

For those who love a sweeter dressing, but want to stick to their ketogenic goals, this recipe is for you! This dressing isn't sweet, per se, but the citrus and tarragon, plus the dressing's creamy texture, satisfy the same cravings. Feel free to adjust the herbs and citrus levels to your tastes.

½ cup mayonnaise

2 tablespoons buttermilk, shaken

2 tablespoons sour cream

Zest and juice of 1 small orange (about ¼ cup juice)

1 to 2 teaspoons sugar-free sweetener of choice (optional)

1 teaspoon dried tarragon

½ teaspoon salt

¼ teaspoon freshly ground black pepper

1 tablespoon poppy seeds

1. In a canning jar or small bowl, combine the mayonnaise, buttermilk, sour cream, orange zest and juice, sweetener (if using), tarragon, salt, and pepper and whisk well.

2. Add the poppy seeds and shake or whisk until well combined and smooth. The dressing will keep covered tightly in the refrigerator for up to 1 week. Shake or whisk again before serving.

MACRONUTRIENTS: 92% Fat, 2% Protein, 6% Carbs

PER SERVING: Calories: 112; Total Fat: 11g; Saturated Fat: 2g; Protein: 1g; Total Carbs: 2g; Fiber: 0g; Net Carbs: 2g

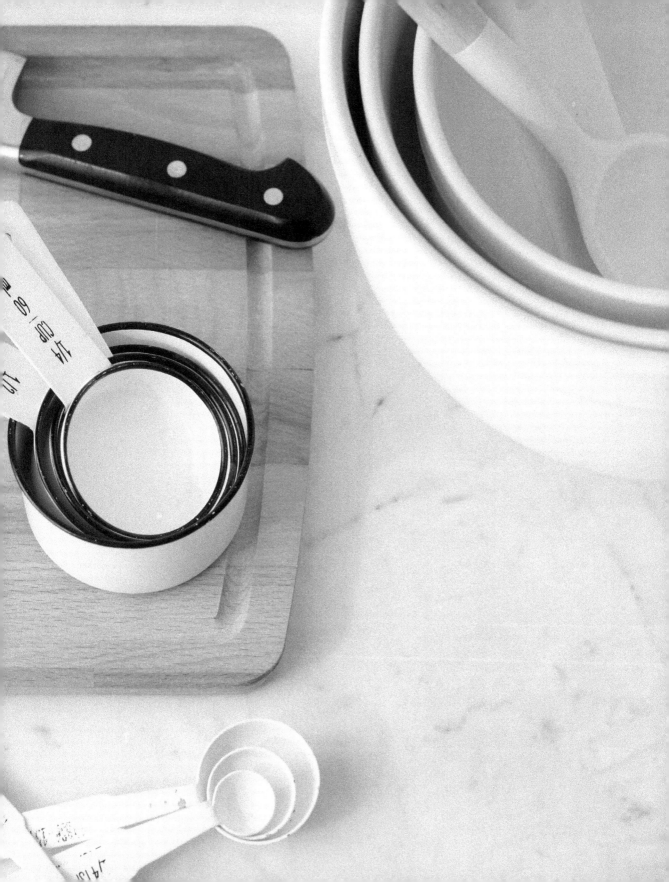

Measurement Conversions

Volume Equivalents	U.S. Standard	U.S. Standard (ounces)	Metric (approximate)
Liquid	2 tablespoons	1 fl. oz.	30 mL
	¼ cup	2 fl. oz.	60 mL
	½ cup	4 fl. oz.	120 mL
	1 cup	8 fl. oz.	240 mL
	1½ cups	12 fl. oz.	355 mL
	2 cups or 1 pint	16 fl. oz.	475 mL
	4 cups or 1 quart	32 fl. oz.	1 L
	1 gallon	128 fl. oz.	4 L
Dry	⅛ teaspoon	—	0.5 mL
	¼ teaspoon	—	1 mL
	½ teaspoon	—	2 mL
	¾ teaspoon	—	4 mL
	1 teaspoon	—	5 mL
	1 tablespoon	—	15 mL
	¼ cup	—	59 mL
	⅓ cup	—	79 mL
	½ cup	—	118 mL
	⅔ cup	—	156 mL
	¾ cup	—	177 mL
	1 cup	—	235 mL
	2 cups or 1 pint	—	475 mL
	3 cups	—	700 mL
	4 cups or 1 quart	—	1 L
	½ gallon	—	2 L
	1 gallon	—	4 L

Oven Temperatures

Fahrenheit	Celsius (approximate)
250°F	120°C
300°F	150°C
325°F	165°C
350°F	180°C
375°F	190°C
400°F	200°C
425°F	220°C
450°F	230°C

Weight Equivalents

U.S. Standard	Metric (approximate)
½ ounce	15 g
1 ounce	30 g
2 ounces	60 g
4 ounces	115 g
8 ounces	225 g
12 ounces	340 g
16 ounces or 1 pound	455 g

REFERENCES

Campos, H., J. J. Genest, Jr., E. Blijlevens, et al. "Low Density Lipoprotein Particle Size and Coronary Artery Disease." *Arteriosclerosis and Thrombosis: A Journal of Vascular Biology.* 1992; 12: 187–195. doi.org/10.1161/01.ATV.12.2.187

Chianese, R., R. Coccurello, A. Viggiano, et al. "Impact of Dietary Fats on Brain Functions." *Current Neuropharmacology.* 2018; 16(7): 1059–1085. doi.org/10.2174 /1570159X15666171017102547

Chung, H. Y., D. H. Kim, E. K. Lee, et al. "Redefining Chronic Inflammation in Aging and Age-Related Diseases: Proposal of the Senoinflammation Concept." *Aging and Disease.* 2019; 10(2): 367–382. doi.org/10.14336/AD.2018.0324

D'Abbondanza, M., S. Ministrini, G. Pucci, et al. "Very Low-Carbohydrate Ketogenic Diet for the Treatment of Severe Obesity and Associated Non-Alcoholic Fatty Liver Disease: The Role of Sex Differences." *Nutrients.* 2020 Sep; 12(9): 2748. doi.org/10.3390/nu12092748

Fontana, L., S. Klein, J. O. Holloszy, and B. N. Premachandra. "Effect of Long-Term Calorie Restriction with Adequate Protein and Micronutrients on Thyroid Hormones." *The Journal of Clinical Endocrinology & Metabolism.* 2006, Aug; 91(8): 3232–3235. doi.org/10.1210/jc.2006-0328

Gasior, Maciej, Michael A. Rogawski, and Adam L. Hartman. "Neuroprotective and Disease-Modifying Effects of the Ketogenic Diet." *Behavioural Pharmacology.* 2006 Sep; 17(5–6): 431–439. www.ncbi.nlm.nih.gov/pmc/articles/PMC2367001/

Haskó G., and B. Cronstein. "Regulation of Inflammation by Adenosine." *Frontiers in Immunology.* 2013; 4(85). doi.org/10.3389/fimmu.2013.00085

Jacob, A. "Does Eating a Low-Carb Diet Affect Bowel Movements?" Livestrong.com. October 29, 2018. www.livestrong.com/article/509998-do-low-carbs-affect -bowel-movements/

Kosinski, C., and F. R. Jornayvaz. "Effects of Ketogenic Diets on Cardiovascular Risk Factors: Evidence from Animal and Human Studies." *Nutrients.* 2017 May 19; 9(5): 517. doi.org/10.3390/nu9050517

Masino, S. A., and D. N. Ruskin. "Ketogenic Diets and Pain." *Journal of Child Neurology.* 2013, May. doi.org/10.1177/0883073813487595

Mavropoulos, J. C., W. S. Yancy, J. Hepburn, and E. C. Westman. "The Effects of a Low-Carbohydrate, Ketogenic Diet on the Polycystic Ovary Syndrome: A Pilot Study." *Nutrition & Metabolism.* 2005, Dec. www.ncbi.nlm.nih.gov/pmc/articles /PMC1334192/pdf/1743-7075-2-35.pdf

Mobbs, C. V., J. Mastaitis, F. Isoda, and M. Poplawski. "Treatment of Diabetes and Diabetic Complications with a Ketogenic Diet." *Child Neurology.* 2013 Aug; 28(8): 1009–1014. doi.org/10.1177/0883073813487596

Vidali, S., S. Aminzadeh, B. Lambert, et al. "Mitochondria: The Ketogenic Diet–A Metabolism-Based Therapy." *International Journal of Biochemistry & Cell Biology.* 2015 Jun; 63: 55–59. doi.org/10.1016/j.biocel.2015.01.022

Wlodarek, D. "Role of Ketogenic Diets in Neurodegenerative Diseases (Alzheimer's Disease and Parkinson's Disease)." *Nutrients.* 2019 Jan; 11(1): 169. doi.org/10.3390/nu11010169

Wood, R. J., J. S. Volek, Y. Liu, et al. "Carbohydrate Restriction Alters Lipoprotein Metabolism by Modifying VLDL, LDL, and HDL Subfraction Distribution and Size in Overweight Men." *The Journal of Nutrition.* 2006 Feb; 136(2): 384–389. doi.org/10.1093/jn/136.2.384

INDEX

ACKNOWLEDGMENTS

For my beautiful and giving parents. Thank you for always supporting me in all my endeavors and teaching me the importance of good food enjoyed with good people. I am one lucky lady to have been raised by you!

As always, I am grateful for my clients who are strong inside and out. You are the inspiration behind this book and the reason I love what I do. Each and every one of these recipes was developed with you in mind and I hope you enjoy them!

I also want to thank my editor, Cecily McAndrews, and the fantastic team at Callisto Media who make the writing process seamless and fun. I am grateful to have had you by my side during this project.

ABOUT THE AUTHOR

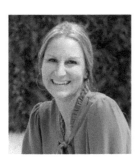 **Molly Devine** is a registered dietitian who specializes in digestive health, healthy weight management, and chronic disease prevention through integrative and functional nutrition. She is an advocate for sustainable lifestyle change through nutrition intervention and the founder of MSD Nutrition Consulting, a nutrition counseling and individualized meal-planning service focusing on customized whole foods–based diets for disease prevention and management. She utilizes insurance-based telehealth to work with clients across the country on their health and nutrition goals. Find out more at MSDNutrition.com.

Molly is the author of *Anti-Inflammatory Keto Cookbook*, *Essential Ketogenic Mediterranean Diet Cookbook*, *The Natural Candida Cleanse: A Healthy Treatment Guide to Improve Your Microbiome*; the co-author of *The Ketogenic Lifestyle: How to Fuel Your Best*; and a regular contributor to nutrition-based online media such as *Shape* magazine, Insider, Greatist, HuffPost, *Brides* magazine, and ABC11 *Eyewitness News*.

Molly received her bachelor of science in nutrition sciences from North Carolina Central University and completed her dietetic internship through Meredith College. She also holds a bachelor of science in languages and linguistics from Georgetown University. She lives in Durham, North Carolina, with her family.

CPSIA information can be obtained
at www.ICGtesting.com
Printed in the USA
JSHW050756240521
15044JS00004B/4